Address the Stress

A Relevant Guide to the Oral Systemic Link

Dr. Jill Wade and Dr. Kelly Martin

First published by Dog Ear Publishing
4010 W. 86th Street, Ste H
Indianapolis, IN 46268
www.dogearpublishing.net

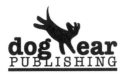

ISBN: 978-145750-714-4

The author, editors, and publisher are not responsible for errors or omissions or for
consequences from application of the book, and make no warranty, expressed or
implied, in regard to the contents of the book. Any practice described in this book
should be applied by the reader in accordance with professional standards of care used
in regard to the unique circumstances that may apply in each situation. The reader is
advised to always check product information and package inserts for changes and new
information regarding dose and contraindications before administering any product.

Printed in the United States of America

Table of Contents

Chapter 8: Relevant Testing and Solutions

Chapter 9: Now Is the Time for the Right Treatment

Chapter 10: Easy Reference to Hormones and Related Organs

Chapter 1
Let's Address the Stress

WE HAVE THE ANSWER TO THE SECRET!
ADRENAL BACKGROUND

Have you ever dreamt of what it would be like to be a queen? If not, stop and think about it for a few seconds. What would you drive, eat and wear? Where would you live? How would you spend your time? How would you feel?

Royalty and the elite feel privy to secrets and information that "normal" people don't have. Kings and queens feel entitled to things that they want. You may not see yourself as royalty, but you are entitled to good health. When it comes to your health, we don't think it is fair to have secrets.

Do you feel exhausted, tired, stressed, and have no energy? If at one point in your life you felt like the life of the party, but now you hardly have enough energy to go to the party, you are not alone. Most people do not fully understand the important influence that long term stress has on your body and the interrelated role that our adrenal glands play in our everyday life. For as bad as you may feel right now, the good news is that with the proper testing, the right treatment, and rest, your stress can be reduced and your adrenals brought back to health. Soon you can begin to feel like your old self again!

Do you have any of these symptoms?

SYMPTOMS:	NONE	MILD	MODERATE	SEVERE
Alcohol intolerance	☐	☐	☐	☐
Allergies and sinus problems	☐	☐	☐	☐
Anxiety	☐	☐	☐	☐
Blood sugar imbalances	☐	☐	☐	☐
Depression	☐	☐	☐	☐
Digestive disorder	☐	☐	☐	☐
Diminished sex drive	☐	☐	☐	☐
Dizziness upon standing	☐	☐	☐	☐
Dry and thin skin	☐	☐	☐	☐
Excessive cravings for sweets	☐	☐	☐	☐
Fatigue	☐	☐	☐	☐
Food and/or inhalant allergies	☐	☐	☐	☐
Hair loss	☐	☐	☐	☐
Headaches	☐	☐	☐	☐
Immune deficiency	☐	☐	☐	☐
Inability to concentrate	☐	☐	☐	☐
Indigestion	☐	☐	☐	☐
Infections (parasitic, bacterial, fungal or viral)	☐	☐	☐	☐
Inflammation	☐	☐	☐	☐
Irritability	☐	☐	☐	☐
Liver, thyroid or pancreatic disorders	☐	☐	☐	☐
Low blood pressure	☐	☐	☐	☐
Low body temperature	☐	☐	☐	☐
Mood swings	☐	☐	☐	☐
Pain in the neck, shoulders & back	☐	☐	☐	☐
Palpitations (heart fluttering)	☐	☐	☐	☐
Poor memory	☐	☐	☐	☐
PMS	☐	☐	☐	☐
Sleep disorders	☐	☐	☐	☐
Weakness/difficulty building muscle	☐	☐	☐	☐
Weight gain/loss	☐	☐	☐	☐

The state of inflammation can ultimately lead to cancer and other serious illnesses such as cardiovascular disease, autoimmune diseases, degenerative diseases, periodontal disease, and accelerated aging. You can see how the magnitude of just one fatigued or exhausted gland can affect so many different areas of health! Visualize the "Circle of Health" again and begin to look at the symptoms in the outer ring to get ideas about which of the inner core jewels may be improperly functioning for you.

The latest wave toward healthcare—the oral systemic link—is a huge example of just how intertwined our entire body is when it comes to stress and inflammation. Many of the above mentioned diseases are defined as CHRONIC INFLAMMATORY DISEASES. Many subtle signs and symptoms of inflammation can be seen inside the mouth.

THE MOUTH IS THE WINDOW TO YOUR HEALTH

A smile should exude confidence, health, and happiness. Perception of your emotional and physical health is influenced by your smile. What does your smile say? If a smile is worth a thousand words, make sure it tells the message you want. Your mouth is the window to your body and it gives many subtle hints to your age, stress level, and overall health. That is why maintaining your oral health is critical.

One of the easiest symptoms to observe in the mouth is STRESS! People just love to clench and grind when they are under a ton of stress. Stress leaves subtle signs like worn teeth, which ages your looks prematurely. A dry mouth or lack of saliva also can occur under chronic stress. Look at your tongue. Is it nice and smooth or does it look like a dried up lake bed with cracks and crevices? Saliva is your body's natural way of protecting itself from cavities. Without enough you will become more susceptible to cavities, infections, and periodontal disease. Everyday science is uncovering more and more direct links of periodontal disease with cardiovascular disease, strokes, and diabetes. You may not be concerned about losing one of your 32 teeth, but when tooth infections affect your one and only heart, you just might change your mind.

HOW DO YOU FATIGUE YOUR ADRENALS?

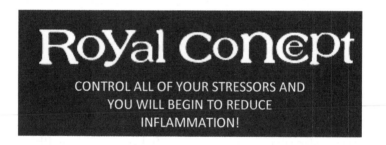

How do you fatigue your adrenals? I know, easy answer right? STRESS! Just live one week of your life. Take that one week and begin to look at it x2 or x10 or x100 weeks. After awhile, the adrenal glands become fatigued or even exhausted simply by the daily stressors of your busy life. Your body is designed so that when the source of immediate stress passes, you can return to a state of rest. When you are constantly in stressful situations, you are constantly on alert. If you do not return to a state of rest, then you risk adrenal fatigue. The cause of fatigue can simply be the stress of daily living, but on top of that stress, add injuries, surgeries, lack of nutrition, lack of rest, or pregnancies and BAM! You have a full on exhaustive episode.

CUT 2 THE CHASE

High stress will decrease your ability to fight infections and absorb nutrients effectively. You may also notice that your allergies are worse in times of stress. Stress which causes high cortisol levels will ultimately lead to adrenal fatigue, which in turn could eventually lead to cancer, cardiovascular disease, autoimmune disease, degenerative diseases, periodontal disease and accelerated aging. The cause of fatigue can simply be stress of daily living, injuries, surgeries, lack of nutrition, lack of rest, pregnancies, etc.

The adrenal glands basically regulate everything, so you must make an effort every day to support their health. You must make these habits a priority of life: sleep, exercise, decreased and controlled stress; support yourself with proper supplements; remove inflammatory foods and remove habits like smoking and excessive alcohol. A proactive and preventive approach to your own mental, physical and dental health will increase your overall health and well-being.

Chapter 2
The "Circle of Health" Philosophy

Our core philosophy centers on the "Circle of Health" and embraces this circle as a map to discovering the best ways of improving our health. The trend in medicine has been specialization. This trend has led to a focus on specific systems and areas of the body. We believe specialization is necessary as long as we do not forget that the body is a WHOLE system and not just a conglomerate of un-connected parts. The body is a fine tuned engine that needs all its pieces to work together to run efficiently. We encourage you to keep reading and keep educating yourself about the systems this concept entails. As you learn more you will eventually begin to be able to help diagnose some of your own medical conditions and support your health care providers in your journey to wellness living.

"CIRCLE OF HEALTH"

Let's get to know our bodies. It's time to learn what makes up the complete system of the human body, what we've called the "Circle of Health." Think of this concept as the royal crown which represents your best life and health. With a crown of a complete golden circle, filled with priceless jewels, you feel like a deserving queen or king.

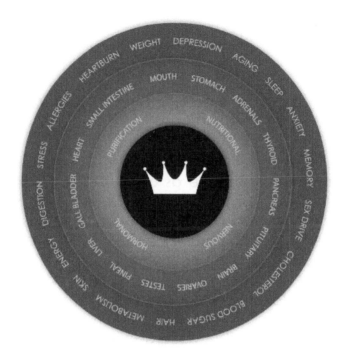

Think of your health as a circle, and within this circle, all of your body's systems are running correctly and efficiently. When this happens you feel great! You feel happy and energetic; you feel like exercising; you find it easier to focus and to work. You don't get sick as often; you sleep well and your libido is healthy. You feel like you want to have sex! If you don't remember the last time you felt good in any of these areas – READ ON! This book was written for you! Just know you are not alone and you are not the only person out there who feels bad.

Let's look at the elements in the "Circle of Health" and review the relevant issues or problems. The inner ring or foundation of the philosophy covers the core elements: hormones, nutrition, purification, nerves. The second ring represents the major organs and systems that compile the core function of staying healthy. The outer ring lists the most common symptoms or problems; these whisper hints to the inner rings.

Mainstream healthcare professionals understand the basics of these systems. However, until you and your provider recognize and honor exactly how intertwined these systems are, your health problems may be misdiagnosed. Many physicians focus on what they are comfortable in addressing and miss other contributing signs and symptoms that also need attention. This is one of the weak links in specialized medicine.

THE FOUR CROWN JEWELS

The core of the "Circle of Health" consists of four basic components. We see each as being a jewel on top of a crown, representing the golden riches of a complete body in a healthy state.

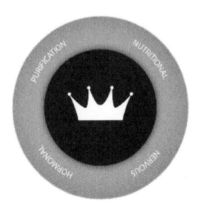

Endocrine System   HORMONES
Digestive System   NUTRITION
Detoxification   PURIFICATION
Nervous System   NERVES

HORMONES – ADDRESS THE STRESS
The simple daily stressors of life can add up to long term chronic stress. This results in the biggest drain to your body's natural hormones. The adrenal gland which is so critical in so many functions of the body is most helpful when supported properly. Remove or control your stressors and support your adrenals and they will back up your sex hormones. Eventually we will all experience a decrease in our sex hormones because, as of today, I have not heard of any Fountain of Youth that will stop the inevitable aging process.

NUTRITION – YOU ARE WHAT YOU EAT
What goes in must come out or get utilized somewhere along the way. Your digestive process starts with the choices you make about what goes in your mouth. Each step along the way of how that food is digested, processed and absorbed is critical. Many organs contribute to the digestive process and, therefore, if only one organ along the way does not function properly, then you may not be getting the fuel you think you are. Surprisingly enough, our digestive track creates 60% of our body's immune system; therefore, it is critical when dealing with allergies, diabetes, and autoimmune diseases to look closely at your entire digestive tract.

PURIFICATION – ARE YOU INFLAMMED?
Inflammation is a key that unlocks so many secrets to the destructive disease process. The act of inflammation seems to link many oral and systemic diseases together. The way cells react to toxins leads them to progress towards cancer, cardiovascular disease, periodontal disease, and increase the aging process. Preventive purification steps can lead to an overall healthier life.

NERVES – THE CURVE IN YOUR HIGHWAY

Your body is an intricate highway of nerves that regulate your entire function consciously and unconsciously. If you have or create an obstacle in that road, you may find yourself on a curving, downward path to poor health. Keeping your physical body supported by good bone and healthy muscles will enable your nervous system to respond to your body's needs.

PRINCESS ALLIE'S STORY

Let's take a moment to introduce you to Princess Allie, a young woman full of vibrant energy, good looks, and a zest for life. Her crown jewels or core components to her health are in good shape and functioning effectively. Princess Allie has a sleek well-toned muscular body that radiates to others that she is healthy. Her beautiful locks of hair, bright eyes and terrific smile illuminate to all that she is happy and confident. Her time is spent energetically dancing to a fun rhythm of life.

Her bodily system consists of strong muscles, bone, and nerves that send clear and fast messages from her brain to her organs and well functioning systems. Her active lifestyle helps to keep her core functioning effectively.

Hormones are in abundance for this princess searching for her prince charming. She is in her prime reproductive years of a well-balanced life.

Now nutritionally Princess Allie eats whatever she wants, with no worries about her weight. The buffet of her life includes poor nutritional value decisions, and she also feasts of fine wines to assure she is the life of the party. This leads to the start of some detoxification and prediabetic issues, but because the majority of her core systems are functioning properly, within hours she can recover from a fantastic night at the ball.

THE ORGANS OR SYSTEMS

Let's look at the circle that lists the organs of your body:

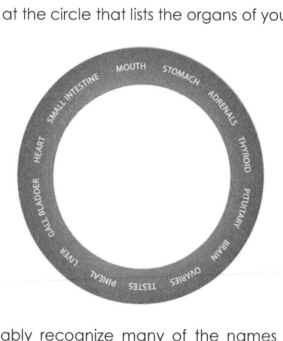

You probably recognize many of the names of these organs and have possibly dealt with a few specific ones in your past health history. Someone in your family has probably had an issue with one of these systems, which is why your family history plays a part in your health. Like it or not, we are turning into our mothers!

Our genetic makeup is passed down to us from the DNA of our parents. This is something that must be taken into consideration. Don't fight it. The information you learn from their history is a gift they have given you.

You should research and understand their problems or issues, be proactive in taking concrete steps to address their relevance to your health, and keep yourself healthier than you would be without this family history at your disposal.

QUEEN ISABELLA'S STORY

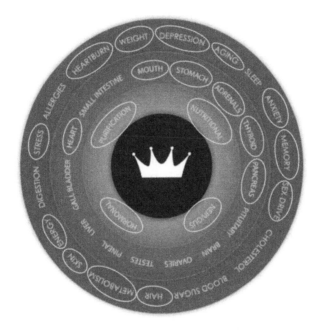

Consider that a royal blood line has been mapped out to you for generations, just as Queen Isabella's has been.   This queen's family history has seen much pollution, so Queen Isabella was not surprised when she began to have the issues with her heart and her back that her father the king had experienced.

This constant problem has lead her path to bone loss, osteoporosis, and loss of much of her muscle mass—the last because she hasn't exercised due to constant pain and arthritis. Her nervous system no longer contributes to her health. The pathway to her nerve impulses is blocked and yet hyperactive in other areas. Her joints and arteries are in a state of inflammation.

Queen Isabella, no longer of childbearing years, has reached menopause and lacks many of her natural hormones.

For 50 years she has ruled her kingdom well, but her days of multiple major decisions have brought her seemingly endless stress. Her adrenals are exhausted and no longer back up her sex hormones or thyroid. She's lost the desire to get out of her palace for a walk or a coach ride to the opera. Pain and fatigue now overrule her social life.

The once strong and vibrant queen now seems replaced with a less social, more irritable, tired-looking queen. Her body is frail and bended, her hair thin and gray, and her face wrinkled and stern. She now passes for a stoic when once she exuded frolicsome gaiety.

Nutritionally the queen could eat literally anything she wanted, but she instead settles for a much smaller meal of carbohydrates, sugars, and salt. She no longer enjoys eating because of the heartburn and digestive issues she uncomfortably experiences.

The queen's recent battle with thyroid cancer revealed that her lifestyle of high stress, poor nutrition, and no exercise only encourages the toxicity that turns healthy cells into cancerous ones.

Queen Isabella does have hope. As royalty, she has the means to get sound health care advice so she can get back on track to living her best life. Finding her balance will be essential as she puts together a successful plan to slow down the effects of aging.

THE SYMPTOMS

Let's focus on the third ring of the "Circle of Health." As you can see, in this circle you will find a myriad of symptoms. As health care providers this is what we deal with every day – symptoms. Patients do not come in complaining that their pancreas hurts or that they feel their ovaries no longer producing estrogen.

Instead we providers have to take the time to listen to the hints your body is telling us via your symptoms. We can either take the time to observe the whispers or just write you a script for a magic pill to cover up the issue until it decides to scream at you.

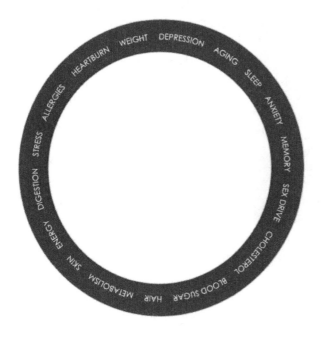

So many symptoms get overlooked and unnoticed. Many times you do not even realize they are all closely linked together, so you do not even mention them to your doctors. Well, do yourself a favor and STOP that thought process. Symptoms are important. Nobody knows your body better than you do. STOP and listen to what your body is trying to tell you. And then share that information!

Have you ever had this happen to you? You went on a diet that you followed step by step? You organized your meal list, went to the grocery store, packed your lunch every day and followed the diet precisely. You deprived yourself of things you wanted and spent a lot of time and energy to achieve the results you desired. You anxiously approach the scale to see how much weight you've dropped, but the number that shows up is actually two pounds more than when you started!?!? How awful! You are frustrated and your inner voice

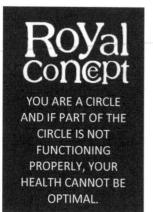

begins to scream and to tell you just how foolish you were to ever think that this diet would work. Within a week you are off the diet, stuffing your face with chocolate because chocolate = LOVE!

Let's throw out a quick explanation of this scenario. If your body has been in an unhealthy state for some time, your system or "Circle of Health" could be out of sync. Your inability to lose weight is a huge scream from your body telling you that core elements to your health are not functioning. You could have a hormonal imbalance, a malfunctioning thyroid, an absorption issue in your small intestine, or you could be eating the wrong type of foods for your blood type.

Considering your body as a whole is how you should approach dieting. If you are in a state of adrenal exhaustion and stress, there is no diet in the world that is going to allow you to lose weight. Your body is in survival mode and it is not going to allow itself to give up anything because it thinks it might need it. You and your check book are much better off approaching and relieving your underlying health issues first and then begin your new diet and exercise plan.

DUCHESS RACHEL'S STORY

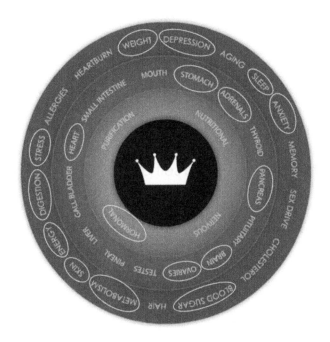

Let's introduce you to the Duchess Rachel. She rules her busy palace full of servants and children. Daily life is full of activity, decisions, frustrations, and glimmers of occasional joy.

You'd expect her active lifestyle to lead her to physical fitness, but instead she has put on over 40 pounds; and no matter what she does, she cannot get it off. She wants to exercise but no longer has the energy or motivation to do so. Her muscles are beginning to atrophy, and her hips and waist, since she bore children, seem to hold most of her weight.

The duchess finds herself much more anxious than ever before; she worries unceasingly about all the details and people in her life. She stays up at night unable to fall asleep, her mind full of details, encounters, and upcoming events. Sometimes she awakens suddenly to a bout of hot flashes.

All of this points directly to her state of pre-menopause. When Duchess Rachel puts herself first for a couple of weeks and rests, eats well-balanced meals, takes supplements and optimizes her lifestyle, she begins to find her balanced wellness state of living. But with her busy schedule, she too easily looses the momentum and goes right back to her old self again.

When she is at the top of her game, she is one beautiful example of strong, successful royalty. But when she is down you can see it in her eyes, skin color and tone, and lack of smile.

CUT 2 THE CHASE

It's time, right now, to address your stress in light of the "Circle of Health" concept. While this book cannot cover all the details of each system and symptom, we hope it will at least increase your awareness that they all have influence on each other. Become more aware of your own body telling you subtle hints to your underlying health concerns by listening to your symptoms. Help find the missing piece or "Crown Jewel" of your circle by sharing information with your health care providers. No one knows your body better than you. As you keep reading, feel good in knowing that you are not going crazy. All of your symptoms are real, and there are real reasons making you feel the way you do.

The stories of Princess Allie, Duchess Rachel, and Queen Isabella are shared in hopes of giving you some visuals of how symptoms are inter-related and what they may look like. Stop now and listen to your body. What is it whispering to you? What is it shouting?

_____
_____
_____
_____

Circle whichever symptoms, systems, or core issues you are experiencing.

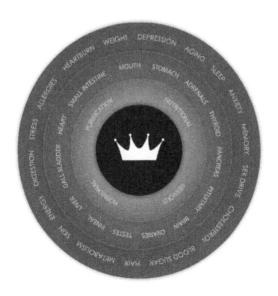

Chapter 3
What Happened to Your Groove?

INTRODUCTION: ABOUT STRESS & IDENTIFYING THE STRESSORS

Think back to the days of your youth when you had energy, a good figure, and best of all—your groove! Remember getting ready for a night out with the girls at 7 o'clock, even though the party did not begin until 10 o'clock?

Tunes rocked in the background, and the rhythm of life was upbeat as you laughed and carried on while teasing, crimping or curling your luscious locks. Not to mention how many outfits you tried on and threw on the floor, only to finally find the perfect one that showed off your smoking hot body in all the right places.

You would dance the night away and be shocked to hear the shouting of "last call" over the music, a sign the night was almost over. How could it be 2:00 o'clock already? We just got here, and we're dominating the dance floor!

After a little more partying at home and a few Cheetos, you finally turned in for the night--or morning. The next morning, or afternoon, came around complete with a parched mouth, headache and desperate need for a Whataburger with a side of Advil.

HAVE YOU LOST YOUR GROOVE?

These days a night out sounds something more like this: scrambling to get the kids where they need to be, doing laundry, cleaning up the kitchen, running to the grocery store for the one item you forgot yesterday, dinner, baths and more laundry!

Huffing and puffing, you realize you need to start getting ready for your date-night out, all of which you are too tired to even think about. You begin to mentally compile the list of all the things you didn't get done today and place them on your "to-do" list for tomorrow. Before you know it, you throw yourself down in the big chair and think to yourself, "Calgon take me away."

The things of your past, like working out, cleaning out the closets and planting flowers, have now been replaced with play-dates, swim lessons and family night at Chick-fil-A. Getting together with your best friend that you haven't seen in weeks seems nearly impossible, even though all you need is a little girl time. You finally have a date-night planned, and so the getting ready process begins; but this time around, it's a little different than when you were in your twenties.

You take baby steps into the shower and say, "Can I get by without shaving my legs? Really it's been only a week–better shave them just in case someone brushes up against me by accident!"

You hop out and lay on the bed stark naked under the fan so you can quit sweating long enough to put on your lotion, deodorant and delicates. On your way to the closet you see out of the corner of your eye the bagel that you had for breakfast now permanently sitting on your waist. With a big sigh and a quick prayer, you begin to pick out an outfit for the evening.

Choosing an outfit is not as much fun as it used to be, mostly because nothing fits and/or the best of your wardrobe was in style last decade.

In the end, you try on as many clothes as you used too, but now you're trying to figure out how to hide some of your assets rather than flaunt them! Finally, you've gotten dressed in your "go to" black dress and reach for the only thing that still looks good on you— a great pair of shoes!

As you make your way to the door to escape, you detour to kiss the kids who squirm under the foreign touch of your lipstick. They say "Mommy, is that you?" With a glimmer of hope that your groove is coming back you drive away in the mini-van happy to be free. Free! Even if only for a few hours! Wow, it's only 7:10 and you are on your way. You're only 25 minutes late compared to your normal 30 to 40 minutes. A couple of drinks later, when your shoes are cutting off your circulation and your Spanx are riding up and down, you look at your watch and think, "How in the world is it only 10 o'clock? It's past my bedtime! The kids will wake up at 8am regardless of how late I'm up." You decide to forego the after-dinner cocktails for pajama pants and a t-shirt.

How did you get here? Where did you go? When did you lose your groove? And, the most important question, how can you get it back?

The first step to getting back into your little black dress is to address the stress. Stress comes in many forms and over time takes a toll on us all. We all feel the aches and pains of chronic stress. Many people deny that they are stressed because they mistakenly equate being stressed to being unhappy.

Happiness has nothing to do with stress. You can be very happy in life and relationships and still be stressed "to the max." Take a deep breath and relax while you read the rest of this chapter, and answer the questions at the end to see if you are truly experiencing the signs of stress. Admitting that you are stressed doesn't make you a bad person; quite the contrary, it makes you normal!

There are many different forms of stress. We are going to allow you to pinpoint the stress in your life. At the end of each section, score how many stressors you have within each category. At the end, you will add up your stress factors.

CARE TAKING

New Baby = New Stress
That bundle of joy that you just brought home is a wonderful blessing that comes complete with a bundle of stress! Sleeplessness and interrupted sleep can weaken even the strongest and healthiest parents. Everything is new and different and keeps you on edge day in and day out. The guilt you feel about going back to work and leaving the baby is mentally exhausting. You are on a hormonal roller coaster ride that depletes your body of normal functioning actions and thoughts.

Older Children = Old Stress
As the kids grow you realize that the troubles and hard times you faced in the past were small issues. Now that the kids have grown, so has the stress they can cause.

Keeping up with who needs to be where and at what time, and with all the school and extra-curricular activities, can feel like you are doing the job of a full-time event planner, minus the pay and days off work.

Illness of a Loved One
A family member who is ill creates a stressful situation that weighs heavily on your heart. Taking care of his or her needs can be as demanding mentally as it is physically. You feel sadness and worry watching a loved one suffer. Caretaking often requires lifting and moving, and these take a toll on your body.

Keeping up with doctor appointments and the details regarding medications, tests, etc. is a full-time job and responsibility. Older family members may add additional stress—they can be much harder to deal with than younger children. The young children are used to being told what to do, while the adults aren't and sometimes don't want to do what's best for them and aren't shy about telling you about their physical discomfort and frustration with your suggestions.

Sickness
If you have recently had surgery or been stricken by an illness, even though you might be feeling better, you still need time to heal. The stress of healing is significant, although not always recognizable; your own care is usually rushed and overlooked.

Preventive wellness living has to be the goal. Anything less is a stress on your body whether or not you recognize poor health.

In the lines below, write the health issues you are dealing with (e.g. hormone imbalances, menopause, allergies, arthritis, blood pressure issues, diabetes, periodontal issues). Include any illness or issues in your family history.

_____

_____

_____

_____

_____

Work as a Care Giver

If your career is all about care, then you may find yourself tapped of extra energy at the end of a work day. Some people choose a form of care giving as a career. Over time, working in this profession can cause you to store a great deal of sympathy. Compassion fatigue is a serious issue that is getting more research and attention every day. Some examples of jobs in the care giving industry are doctors, nurses, child or elderly care workers, and teachers.

Now go grab a pen and answer the following questions about your **caretaking** responsibilities:

RESPONSIBILITIES OF A CARETAKER

New Baby # of Kids (ages 2 and under): _____ x 3 = _____
Children # of Kids (ages 2 -7): _____ x 1 = _____
Older Children # of Kids (ages 7-15): _____ x 2 = _____
Illness of a Loved One # of sick family _____ x 2 = _____
members:
Sickness Recently had surgery or stricken
by illness, still recovering.   +3 = _____
Terminal Illness You are battling a serious
illness with no definite solution in the near   + 5 = _____
future:
Caregiver If your occupation is care giving: + 5 = _____
TOTAL CARETAKING POINTS: _____

TIME

Full-time job
Working 9 to 5, or does it seem more like 8 to 6? When the alarm clock starts to beep, are you already counting down the minutes until you can get back in bed? The stress associated with some jobs is enough to make you pull the covers over your head and hide. Some jobs are more physical and stressful than others.

To work or not to work
Staying at home with children and running a house-hold is a full-time job. Let's not overlook this job! It is probably one of the hardest, albeit most rewarding, on earth. If you are a stay-at-home parent, you have as much stress (if not more) than someone who works outside of the home.

2nd job to make ends meet
Not only do you have one job, but you have taken a second job to make ends meet. That is definitely more stress and less time to take care of every day responsibilities and rest.

Owning your own business
For all the wonderful things owning your own business may offer, there are always many stressors associated with it. The more employees you have, the more stress. You feel not only responsible for yourself, but also for each of the employee's families. If you or your spouse own your own business or you both do, add points to your account.

Unemployed
The way today's economy is going, you could look up and find yourself unexpectedly out of work. After you wake up from the initial shock, you begin your new

journey of possibilities. The new options in front of you can be exhilarating, yet the process can also be rather stressful.

Answer the following questions about your **time**:

YOUR TIME

Work full-time:	+ 4 = _____
Work part-time:	+ 2 = _____
Full-time stay-at-home parent:	+ 4 = _____
Part-time parent:	+ 2 = _____
If you have a second job:	+ 4 = _____
Own your own business:	+ 8 = _____
Spouse owns own business:	+ 4 = _____
Unemployed:	+ 3 = _____
TOTAL TIME POINTS:	_____

RELATIONSHIPS

A spouse, a partner, a significant other and children are all relationships that require time and attention. Close relationships with family and siblings are time-consuming, but all play an important role as strength and support for you.

On the flip side, the time and effort it takes to work through a bad relationship is even worse and more time-consuming.

Spouse
"Till death do us part"! Sometimes death seems easier. This partnership in life can potentially bring you so much joy and love, or it can be a huge reason why you feel so bad. Love is a powerful healer, but without it, there can be a void that nothing else can fill. Not even chocolate cake! Be aware of your relationship and its boundaries.

Children

A place deep within your heart can be filled with the special gift of having a child. But I think we can all agree that from the time they arrive they do add a big increase in your stress level.

Thank goodness it is natural to want to have children—why else would we choose to intentionally encounter so much stress.

Family

Parents: They are in our DNA. We are a part of them no matter how much we love them or hate them

In-Laws: Need I say more? For those of you that get along, more power to you. Feel blessed.

Siblings: Brothers and sisters can bring up a wide range of emotional baggage. But without a doubt the more you have the more drama potential there is in the family dynamic.

Answer the following questions regarding your **relationships**:

RELATIONSHIPS

Spouse or Serious Relationship	+ 4 = _____	
# of Children you have	_____ + 3 = _____	
# of Living Parents	_____ + 2 = _____	
# of In-Laws	_____ + 1 = _____	
# of Siblings	_____ + 2 = _____	
# Bad/Unhealthy Relationships:	_____ x 2 = _____	

TOTAL RELATIONSHIP POINTS: _____

COMMITMENTS

There are only 24 hours in a day, and you should be sleeping at least 8 hours. That only leaves 16 hours a day to get things done. Now do you see why you feel so stressed out and tired? How much of your day is taken up by commitments?

Give yourself a point for each activity you are committed to weekly or bi-weekly. Examples are: local women's leagues, church committees, kid's school activities and support groups, or monthly group outings such as book clubs or bunko.

Write down your list of commitments (1 point each):

_____
_____
_____
_____
_____
_____
_____
_____
_____
_____
_____
_____
_____
_____
_____
_____
_____
_____
_____

TOTAL COMMITMENT POINTS: _____

FINANCIAL COMMITMENTS

Financial stress can be (and usually is) the worst of all stressors. If you are in debt or are barely making it by living paycheck to paycheck, financial stress can be a constant drain to your attitude and health.

Credit card debt is a big hurdle that most Americans face. Stop rewarding yourself with <u>things,</u> and instead reward yourself by feeling better because you are working towards a goal of financial freedom. About 43% of American families spend more than they earn each year. The average household carries over $10,000 in credit card debt!

FINANCIAL COMMITMENTS
If you are in debt (add 1 point for
each $5,000 you owe):   = _____
If you have filed for bankruptcy
recently (within 3 years):   x 10 = _____
TOTAL FINANCIAL POINTS: _____

Are you ready to add up all your stress factors and get a realistic view of how much stress you are encountering each and every month?

STRESS FACTORS

Caretaking:	_____
Time:	_____
Relationships:	_____
Time Commitments:	_____
Financial Commitments:	_____

TOTAL STRESS FACTORS: _____

RESULTS

If your points fall in these ranges, we feel you are experiencing these levels of stress.

25 points or fewer:
Sparkle: You have one or two small things that create some stress in your life.

26-45 points:
Bling: You may have only a few items that cause you stress, but these few things have some oomph!

46-65 points:
Glitter: You are starting to get some glimmer of too many things going on, and you are beginning to feel overwhelmed and scattered.

66 points or more:
Be-Dazzled: Girl, you have got way too much happening! You are wearing yourself out...You need to learn how to say "NO!"

Now that you're stressed out from reviewing your stress, I bet we have your attention! Get excited because there is HOPE! We are going to give you direction on how to get back to living and feeling well!

Chronic, long-term stress will slowly rob your body of essential elements it needs. Some people can handle this level of stress for a long time until the natural effects of aging begin to catch up with them.

There is hope if you are feeling bad. You can control or remove some of the stressors you just identified. You can rebuild your adrenals, rest and re-set your metabolism via nutrition and hormonal supplements. Begin to treat yourself like the Queen that you are. You are entitled to feel your best; now let's get you there!

CUT 2 THE CHASE

The first step to feeling your best is to begin treating yourself like a queen. Queens are rarely stressed, so we suggest you begin your focus and attention there. This chapter's main focus was to make sure you understood that you do have stress in your life. The rest of the book focuses on educating you about what stress does to your body and how to counter-balance the effects of long-term stress.

Come back later to this chapter and your lists and spend some time deciding if you need to address problem areas of your life more seriously. Perhaps you need to practice saying "No" more often. Seeking a good counsel for poor relationships or financial issues might be a smart move on your part. Trusted counsel to your overall health may also be needed to address adequately any deeper stressors.

If you are not satisfied with your life, then maybe go back to school or consider a job change. When you begin to take back control of your life and address the stress, you will feel like a queen again!

Chapter 4
"The Day in the Life of a Hormone"

PLAY BY PLAY

None of us wants to live the sad, dull life of Bill Murray's character in *Groundhog Day*, over and over again without end. We want to live life to the fullest.

We want *you* to have an Oprah "Aw ha!" moment. To do so you need to understand in better detail exactly what your hormones *are* or *are not* doing for you. Enjoy this day in the life story of what your hormones really do on a daily basis!

SUNRISE

Beep! Beep! Beep! Click. Yawn, stretch and sigh. Her Majesty awakens for another glorious day with her royal subjects.

At the end of a wonderful night of REM sleep, you feel like sleeping beauty. The adrenal glands kick into gear to provide cortisol to gently get the body ready for activity and to increase metabolism. Epinephrine is produced to quicken the heart rate and narrow blood vessels for standing. Because you didn't eat all night, the liver is producing glycogen, which breaks down glucose stored in your liver and muscles.

After a healthy breakfast, carbohydrates break down into glucose and the pancreas starts pumping out insulin to get the glucose into the cells for energy. Hormones in the gastrointestinal tract are increasing mobility and secretions, and causing the gallbladder to release stored bile to help break down fats. In summary, you truly feel like a queen!

DAYTIME

A queen makes many decisions during the day that will cause the adrenal glands to produce cortisol and adrenaline, depending on the type of stress. Confrontation will usually cause the fight or flight response, which will require a large excretion of adrenaline. Working out during the day will cause cortisol and epinephrine to peak in response, causing heart rates and respirations to soar, increasing metabolism and fat loss.

Endorphins kick in and elevate the mood and dampen aches and pains. During exercise, the heart secretes atrial natriuretic peptide, which signals the kidneys to produce salty urine. This also inhibits the adrenal glands' production of aldosterone, which helps to maintain blood pressure by controlling fluid flow in the kidneys. This is why exercise creates the need to urinate.

After exercise, blood sugar and insulin are low. This, in turn, causes hunger. A snack in the sunshine will cause the production of cholecalciferol, which is then converted to vitamin D. Vitamin D helps the body use calcium. If blood calcium drops a bit, then the parathyroid gland secretes parathyroid hormone, drawing calcium from the bones. By eating a calcium rich snack, the parathyroid will release calcitonin, which will deposit calcium back into the bones.

SUNSET

At the end of the day, a hot flash is triggered by the deficiency of estrogen. Blood surges to the surface of the skin, heart rate and breathing quicken, and sweating begins. This can happen during pre-menopause as well as menopause. (More estrogen is needed during times of stress).

These changes stimulate the part of the brain that controls body temperature and are synchronized with core temperature. Late afternoon and early evening are prime times for hot flashes. The thyroid has been working steadily all day to control metabolism. If the body gets cold and shivers, then the thyroid will secrete more of its hormones to increase metabolism and generate internal warmth.

Sex causes a production of cortisol and epinephrine in response to the physical exertion. Feel-good endorphins are released and oxytocin is triggered during orgasm. Oxytocin produces uterine contractions during labor, but also plays a role in sexual arousal.

NIGHTTIME

At bedtime, the pineal gland secretes melatonin. This light-sensitive hormone helps regulate the body's circadian rhythm. All in all, it's enough to exhaust any average duchess. Now off to a restful night's sleep fit for a queen, preferably on 1,000 or higher thread-count sheets.

CUT 2 THE CHASE

If that is a day in the life of a hormone for most women in a pre-menopause situation, what can we learn about the dos and don'ts of the day?

Here are just a few life lessons to put into your daily routine of addressing the stress:

- Achieving REM sleep, a deeper and more restful, healing sleep, will allow you to start your day off right.

- Eating a low glycemic, high protein breakfast will help control insulin and cortisol.

- Minimizing stress throughout the day keeps cortisol low and inhibits insulin resistance, thereby keeping your mid-section thin.

- Stress increases cortisol and insulin, increasing the need for glucose. The carbohydrate cravings set in so intensely you feel you must eat CARBS.

- Exercising even 10 to 15 minutes a day will help achieve good overall health with minimal effort. In other words, a little exercise goes a long way in maintaining your well-being.

- Have sex. It's fun and it produces some incredible health benefits.

- Go to bed at a reasonable time. Ideally, no later than 10 p.m. Aim to get a minimum of eight hours of good, deep, restful sleep to start you off right on the new day ahead. Going to bed later allows the cortisol levels to start to rise again, which you experience as getting a second wind. In this scenario, you are not letting your adrenals rest in order to heal and replenish so they can function at full steam ahead on the days to come. In short, a second wind today will take the wind out of your sails tomorrow!

Chapter 5
You Are What You Eat!

Chronic stress eventually influences your nutrition. It can lead to strong food cravings, the need for caffeine jump-starts, and an unhealthy digestive tract that negatively influences your immune system.

Your body is an amazing piece of machinery that needs the proper fuel to go anywhere. If you feed yourself the cheapest fuel available (junk food), then expect your engine to eventually stop working. For those of you who work hard at feeding yourself all the right things, keep reading!

If you have tried to lose that same 10 pounds multiple times just to put it right back on again, then maybe it is time to step back and have some testing done to make sure your body is functioning properly, rather than just beginning that next fad diet. Even if you practice the all organic or vegan life, you might be having the same problems the rest of us "junk food junkies" are having.

Once again, your body is a closed system: remember the "Circle of Health." If your hormones or organs cannot support your body's metabolism properly, then it does not matter what you place in your mouth. You still may not be able to lose weight. This is why dieting can be so hard and frustrating. A few simple tests may reveal what part of your engine needs some maintenance.

DO YOU HAVE A SIX PACK OR A MUFFIN TOP?

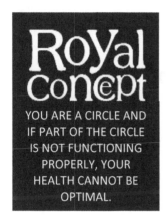

YOU ARE A CIRCLE AND IF PART OF THE CIRCLE IS NOT FUNCTIONING PROPERLY, YOUR HEALTH CANNOT BE OPTIMAL.

It is common to see individuals who don't seem to be overweight, yet who have excess fat around their hips, thighs or waist. In fact, these people may be slender except for those "problem" areas.

For those of you that have a muffin top problem, perhaps it is from high levels of cortisol or stress. Elevated cortisol causes insulin resistance, which increases the likelihood of your body storing sugar as fat. The relationship between cortisol and fat storage is why several weight loss systems have focused on cortisol and controlling its effects.

CRAZY CARBOHYDRATE CRAVINGS

Many times when you are stressed, fatigued, and tired your hypothalamus will begin to play tricks on you and tell you that you need things. Stress increases cortisol and insulin, therefore increasing the need for glucose. The carbohydrate cravings are so intense you feel you <u>must</u> have some. What is the number one source of glucose? CARBS!

WHAT IS INSULIN RESISTANCE?

No, it is not some new diet that makes you want to resist all sugars. Sorry. It is what happens to your body after feeding yourself exactly what you crave anytime you want. Food is typically absorbed into the bloodstream in the form of sugars. An increase in sugar in the bloodstream signals the pancreas to increase the secretion of insulin. If you eat a big piece of chocolate cake, insulin is pumped into the blood stream to handle all the sugar. This hormone attaches to cells, removing sugar from the bloodstream so that it can be used for energy.

Insulin resistance occurs when a normal amount of insulin is not able to begin the process. In response, the body secretes even more insulin in an attempt to maintain normal blood sugar levels (hyper-insulin-emia). Insulin resistance is the first stage of Type II diabetes.

If you are a diabetic, then it's more than likely your adrenals are exhausted because they support the pancreas that controls insulin, as we saw in the "Circle of Health".

Royal Concept

Dietary changes like eating foods with higher fiber and lower glycemic indexes, along with moderate exercise, reduce the risk of Type II diabetes.

The first treatment of insulin resistance is to encourage lifestyle modifications with weight loss as the goal. Exercising a minimum of 2 ½ hours a week reduces the risk of Type II diabetes. Lifestyle changes trump medication. A magic pill might be only masking the problem long term. It surely is not correcting the underlying health issues.

Dietary modifications like increasing fiber and eating foods with a lower glycemic index is essential in managing blood sugar levels. Last but not least, decreasing stress will contribute to keeping the body's insulin levels regulated.

CHEW ON THIS

The mouth is the gateway for your entire nutritional system. Proper digestion begins with chewing; therefore, keeping your teeth functioning properly and without pain and infection could literally add more years to your life. Be smart about your oral health, it is no coincidence that we have "Wisdom teeth."

When you properly chew your food and it mixes with saliva, the digestive process has already begun by the time it reaches your stomach. Critical levels of proper acids in your stomach continue the process.

Acid reflux, better known as heart burn is a huge sign that your body is deficient or working improperly. It could also be a big red flag to STRESS.

Hydrochloric acid, the key strong acid to digesting food, needs to stay in your stomach. If it is released back up the pipes it can do damage to your teeth and create an environment for bacteria that promote cavities and inflammation.

While we are on the subject matter of acids, let's discuss PH levels. Did you know that the foods you eat can contribute to your body's natural ph balance? A diet high in certain foods can increase your acidity level overall, while a more alkaline diet can lower it. Consider educating yourself more on specific food ph levels if you are having health concerns in this area.

Food sensitivities are also an area of concern when discussing the digestive track. If you develop food sensitivities, then your immune system may be at an optimal level.

THE THREE C's

Does your highness enjoy the pleasures of life? What we call the three C's?

Carbohydrates!
Chocolate!
Cokes!

Join the crowd. At times, it is nearly impossible not to hear and to succumb to the Three C's calling. Cravings are your body's signal that you are probably deficient in some specific nutrient or that your endocrine system is not working effectively.

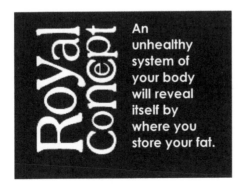

Royal Concept

An unhealthy system of your body will reveal itself by where you store your fat.

When you feed yourself the proper foods and you actually absorb them, then you will experience the regal health you deserve. Your body is also telling you something if you keep trying to lose weight and you can't.

We have tried to make this easier to understand by explaining some of the factors that combine and cause you to look and feel the way that you do. Continue to read and see which of the body types you most relate to in this chapter.

MIRROR, MIRROR ON THE WALL

Mirror, mirror on the wall, is my reflection the clue to call? It is hard to look cute in a slinky black dress if your body shape resembles a piece of fruit. Go ahead and look in that full length mirror that you avoid daily to see if you can gain a hint to what might be an underlying reason for your health issues.

Take a few minutes to go look at your body shape in the mirror. See if the shape that reflects is portrayed in one of the following shapes. You may find some clues as to which part of your "Circle of Health" is calling for your attention.

Which shape best describes your body shape?

- Are you a rectangle?

- Are you a square?

- Are you a pear?

- Are you an apple?

WHERE ARE YOUR PROBLEM AREAS?

THE THYROID BODY TYPE

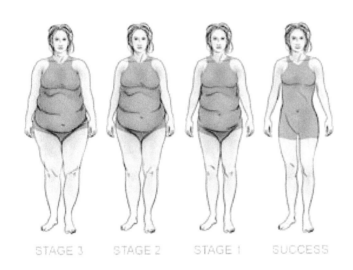

STAGE 3   STAGE 2   STAGE 1   SUCCESS

Primary characteristics:

- Rectangular shape
- Weight gain all over
- Sluggish metabolism
- Spongy fat accumulation

Stage 1:

Noticeable hair loss

Lose outer portion of eyebrows

Loose skin under chin and arms

Stage 2:

> Nails become brittle
>
> Experience constipation
>
> Feet get cold

Stage 3:

> Chronic fatigue
>
> Depression

Cravings:

Since your body has lost the ability to absorb vitamins and nutrients from food, you will crave quick energy carbohydrates such as breads, pasta, sugar, and even alcohol.

Trigger:

No specific triggers.

Symptoms:

You feel you cannot handle stress.
You suffer from exhaustion even though you get plenty of sleep.

Solutions:

Proper testing and supplementation with thyroid hormones

THE ADRENAL BODY TYPE

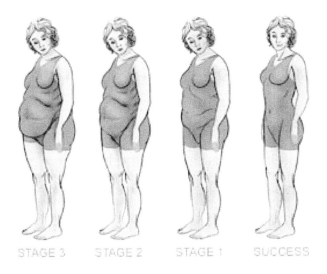

STAGE 3   STAGE 2   STAGE 1   SUCCESS

Primary characteristics:

- Square shaped
- Weight gain as belly fat
- More stress increases cortisol levels
- Fat storage for potential energy
- Active mentally (constantly stressing)

Stage 1:

Dark circles under eyes

Sagging stomach

Face becomes round

Double chin

Fat storage on the back

Stage 2:

> Inflammation
>
> Swollen ankles or hands
>
> Stiffness or pain in hamstrings

Stage 3:

> Muscle protein breaks down in the legs
>
> Arthritis or pain in the heel of the foot/lower back
>
> Twitching under left eye

Cravings:

Chocolate, energy drinks, caffeine, and salt

Trigger:

Caffeine

Symptoms:

Dieting actually makes you worse because it is adding stress to what is already a stressed system.
You feel overwhelmed.

Solutions:

Proper testing for adrenals and then protocol of lifestyle factors such as adequate rest and nutrition. Supplement the adrenal hormones at least four times a day just to stabilize your sugar levels.

THE OVARY BODY TYPE

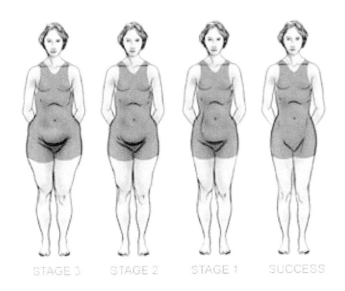

STAGE 3   STAGE 2   STAGE 1   SUCCESS

Primary characteristics:

- Pear shaped
- Weight begins to store as fat below the belly button

Stage 1:

Difficult menstrual cycles with excessive bleeding and pain

Stage 2:

More weight gain in hip area

Cellulite or cottage cheese on thighs and stomach

Upper body stays smaller in relationship to lower body

Waist is still small

Stage 3:

Pain in the tailbone and lower back area

Cravings:

Creamy foods
Dairy
Ice-cream
Cream cheese
Cheese cake
Yogurt

Trigger:

Sugar

Symptoms:

Problems with menstruation is a key symptom to the in-balance between estrogen and progesterone causing fat to accumulate around the ovaries

Solution:

Test hormones and correct deficiencies, most likely progesterone.

THE LIVER BODY TYPE

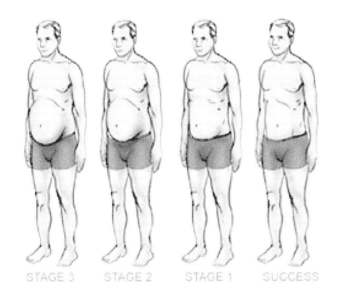

STAGE 3   STAGE 2   STAGE 1   SUCCESS

Primary characteristics:

- Apple shaped
- Most common in men
- "Pot Belly"
- Toxins accumulate in the liver and produce swelling
- With time this swelling turns hard

Stage 1:

Weight gain and protrusion of the gut

Legs stay thin

Stage 2:

> Develop right shoulder pain
>
> Back stiffness in the morning
>
> Sleeping issues causing irritability in the mornings

Stage 3:

> Cravings get worse and demand your meals.
>
> Almost never want vegetables.
>
> The need for nutrition goes beyond simple hunger.
>
> Appetite increases.

Cravings:

Deep fried foods because the liver cannot absorb any fats

Triggers:

No specific triggers.

Symptoms:

Skin irritation
Chronic digestive problems
Whites of eyes are yellowish and bloodshot
Blood pressure and cholesterol will rise to unhealthy level

Solutions:

Wean yourself off of toxins like food and drinks high in preservatives, soft drinks, alcohol, excessive prescriptive drugs.

A liver cleanse is the first line of defense to detoxify the liver

MIRROR, MIRROR ON THE WALL, DO YOU WANT YOUR HEALTH TO FALL?

What should you do? We want you to understand the complexity of your metabolism. It is very important that you be properly tested. You and your health care provider have to take into consideration all the factors in your "Circle of Health" to truly find the answers to your underlying condition.

Think of thorough diagnostic testing results as the crystal ball to your future health and a reflection that makes you look and feel better. Perhaps an underlying thyroid issue will surface that needs drugs to regulate the looping system better, which in turn will increase your metabolism and allow you to finally lose weight. If you look exactly like the adrenal exhausted picture and your test results verify that you are in need of supplements, in no time at all you may finally have the extra energy needed to begin to workout.

DIETING—FAD OR FAB?

Have you lost and gained the same ten pounds several times throughout your life? Let's explore diets for a few minutes. Weight loss is a multi-billion dollar industry. From the years 1980-2000, obesity rates doubled among adults.   About 60 million adults or 30% of the adult population are now obese.

How are you supposed to figure out which diet works best for you? Get ready – it's not a diet – it is a lifestyle change. Until your brain wants to change and you get happy and healthy again, you won't lose weight.   So how do you know what direction to take...what foods are best processed by your body...how to eat right for your blood type? All the choices can make it confusing. Let us just talk about some nutrition basics: absorption, food sensitivities, blood typing, and cravings.

NUTRITIONAL BASICS

Absorption
You can eat all the healthy food you want, take a handful of supplements, and drink lots of water, but if you aren't absorbing enough of the nutrients, then you aren't doing yourself as much as good as you think you are. Most of your absorption takes place in the small intestine, so you want to keep it as healthy as possible and keep inflammation at a minimum. You can do this by knowing what foods you are sensitive to and keeping your micro flora balanced by taking probiotics. If you are suffering from acid reflux or heartburn, you can also take hydrochloric acid and enzymes as your stomach may not be producing enough to properly break down your food. All of these things will contribute to the better absorption of your nutrients.

Food Sensitivities
Most of you have food sensitivities that you are not aware of, and the only way to know for sure is via an

IgG blood test. Sensitivity (IgG) differs from an allergy in that sensitivity will cause symptoms 48-72 hours after ingesting the offending food. An allergic reaction, however, happens immediately.

Think about the movie *Hitch*: Will Smith ate shellfish and his lips and mouth swelled up immediately. After 48-72 hours, most people really can't remember everything they ate that may be causing abdominal pain, diarrhea, skin irritations, hives, or headaches, etc.
In order to decrease general inflammation in your body and to optimize the absorption of nutrients, it's very important to be aware of your food sensitivities. You want to make sure you do not have a "leaky" gut or holes in your small intestine from inflammatory foods. For instance, once you know that gluten is creating some of your severe reactions, you can simply remove it from your diet for 20 days or so. Don't despair, it's not like you can never have it again. Bring it back into your diet slowly and begin a rotational diet. A four-day rotational diet helps you to avoid gaining sensitivities to one main food group.

Blood Typing
Eating for your blood type is certainly worth noting because you should have every advantage when it comes to your health and nutrition.

Some simple basic rules are:

Type A blood types seem to process fruits, grains, and vegetables most efficiently, as well as some fish and fowl, but process red meats the least efficiently.

Type O blood types can get away with being more carnivorous, but don't seem to process grains as well.

The B blood types are a wonderful mixture of the A's and O's.

There is much research on this topic but we wanted to touch on the concept here...just some food for thought, so to speak.

Cravings
Ever wondered why you crave certain foods at certain times? Much of the reason is that your body is telling you that you are deficient in certain nutrients. For example, if you are craving salt, you could be deficient in sodium or iodine; or if you are craving chocolate, you could be deficient in magnesium. Carbohydrate cravings could be your body telling you that you need a quick energy source, due to a poor diet, imbalanced blood sugar or adrenal fatigue. If you are finding yourself having some consistent cravings, then it would definitely be beneficial to find out your deficiencies by having a micronutrient blood test performed. This wonderful test will tell you exactly what you are missing and explain the symptoms you may be experiencing due to the deficiencies.

WHAT IS A LEAKY GUT?

To review, a leaky gut occurs where excessive inflammation in the small intestine from offending foods and toxins creates holes in the surface of the microvillus, the gateway to the bloodstream. These holes allow all sorts of "garbage" into your blood and create a systemic immune response. In other words, it puts your immune system on high alert, to the point that it may start attacking good cells in your body, contributing toward arthritis, psoriasis, etc.

CUT 2 THE CHASE

Adrenal fatigue is caused by chronic stress. Once your body has been under a strain for a long time, body systems begin to shut down and you begin to have difficulty with some or all of the following issues. Your thyroid has to try to make up for the adrenal glands not working and your metabolism falls short. Your cravings increase and absorption issues begin to create the leaky gut situation.   Along with increased levels of cortisol, you begin to put on weight and cannot lose it when you try to diet. When you look in the mirror your shape should give you clues to your underlying health issues. Simply get tested to reveal the problem areas like thyroid or hormone imbalance, high ph balance, diabetes, inflammation, liver toxicity or food sensitivity. Once you begin a protocol for the solutions to the problems, you will begin to function in a more healthy state.

The entire function of your digestive tract, your nutritional choices, your hormone imbalances, and your family history are all key players in your overall immune system.   That is why nutrition is a crown jewel in maintaining your "Circle of Health."

Chapter 6
Where Did My Energy Go?

Has anybody seen my energy? Did I leave it at Starbucks? All kidding aside, do you have just enough energy to get the essential items of the day taken care of, but nothing extra? Do you find yourself doing well until you sit down on the couch and then it's over, you're done, and nothing else is going to happen after that? All these feelings—fatigue, being tired, sleepiness, foggy headedness—are all huge signs of adrenal exhaustion.

Do you ever wake up and feel like you are in the movie *Ground Hog Day*? Another day of the hustle and bustle of life, but you must get up and begin your day while still feeling groggy and tired? If you are not waking up refreshed and ready to rock and roll each day, then you may be drained. Chronic daily stress will begin to deplete you of essential natural elements like hormones and nutrients. As these essential items begin to disappear, you will begin to see more of the symptoms below as a result of their disappearing act.

Decrease in absorption of nutrients
Food cravings
Increase in weight
Increase in irritability
Daily fatigue
Sleep issues
Decrease in saliva

CAFFEINE FIX FOR A SECOND WIND

Do you have every Starbucks, Seven Eleven, and Sonic Happy Hour saved in your GPS? Like a car, do you need to fill up a couple of times a day on caffeine so you don't run out of gas? Do you feel that if it wasn't for caffeine, you might not make it through the day? But what is caffeine really doing for you?

Caffeine is a stimulant that temporarily raises your metabolism and body processes and gives a temporary feeling of energy, but later you crash and burn. Your body craves sugar and carbs for the same reason...you are looking for some quick energy because you are sinking fast.

There is a natural time line to our energy level as it relates to our cortisol production by our adrenal glands. It naturally looks like this: Energy levels are highest in the morning when cortisol peaks after you wake up. By lunchtime you still have energy, but cortisol is about ½ what it was in the morning. By late afternoon, cortisol is about ½ what it was at noon and by bedtime your cortisol has bottomed out, and you are ready to rest.

When you have adrenal fatigue, your cortisol production wanes earlier in the day and you find yourself trying to make up for the decrease in energy by reaching for caffeine and sugar.

WHO HAS TIME OR ENERGY FOR SEX?

When you have adrenal fatigue, you may have no energy for sex and possibly less interest in even thinking about it.

The adrenals also act as an additional producer of your sex hormones (estrogen, progesterone, testosterone). When you are young and your sex organs are fully functioning and you have little to no stress, the adrenals do not have to work very hard. As you age and you have more stress, you need the adrenals to back up your aging and slowing ovaries. But the adrenals may be too busy producing stress hormones like cortisol and adrenaline. In times of stress, reproduction is put on the back burner, so to speak.

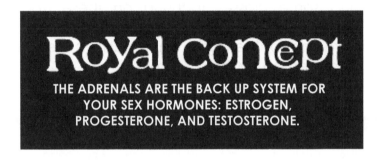

Royal Conept

THE ADRENALS ARE THE BACK UP SYSTEM FOR YOUR SEX HORMONES: ESTROGEN, PROGESTERONE, AND TESTOSTERONE.

WHY DOES EVERYONE SEEM SO CALM AFTER YOGA?

The "Circle of Health" concept is nothing new in the history of healthcare and medicine. Many approaches to medicine focus on the nervous system and how it transmits the information from one area of the body to the next. Chiropractics, acupuncture, massage therapy, and reflexology, just to name a few, have their main focus on keeping the informational highway of our nervous system open for communication.

You can track holistic health and medicine back to ancient times. For example, in ancient Eastern medicine, people placed great focus on chakras, which are "force centers" or whorls of *energy* permeating from a point on the physical body. Chakras are still used today in the practice of yoga. Just as we have broken down different symptoms or areas of the body that are related, these chakras are broken down into seven regions of the body, each related to an endocrine gland that needs to be centered and healthy for overall wellness.

The Eastern medicines took these chakras even further and related them to seven colors of the rainbow and seven musical notes. When you practice yoga, you may find some classes focusing on these colors or humming these particular notes to help center the specific regions of the body. One chakra is the adrenal gland represented by the color red.

Seven CHAKRAS:			
Violet	Top of Head	Pineal Gland	Crown Chakra
Indigo Blue	Center of Forehead	Pituitary Gland	Brow Chakra
Sky Blue	Base of Throat	Thyroid	Throat Chakra
Green	Center of the Chest	Thymus	Heart Chakra
Yellow	Solar Plexus	Pancreas	Solar Plexus Chakra
Orange	Center of Abdomen	Gonads	Orange Chakra
Red	Perineum	Adrenals	Root Chakra

It's interesting how so many years later, health and wellness evidence points in the same direction as it has for so long. These practices have been in place for years because of the health benefits they provide to the human body. Once you begin to focus on the body as a whole, and become more in touch with the different regions of your body, you can then begin to take proactive measures toward being in a place of health. This is the Relevance philosophy based on the main focus of the "Circle of Health."

SUGGESTED STEPS TO A BETTER SITUATION:

- Healthier nutrition choices
- Consistent sleep and rest
- Daily gentle exercise
- Institute a daily time of prayer or meditation
- Begin journey to find answers to health issues with proper testing
- Removal of toxins:
    - People or situations
    - Drugs and alcohol
    - Food preservatives
    - Artificial sweeteners
    - Heavy metals – e.g. lead, mercury, aluminum

CUT 2 THE CHASE

Constant daily stress with no hope for change is a recipe for insanity. You must be willing to put your "glass-slippered" foot down and demand that change be made – first in yourself and second in the people around you. Many sources refer to this as finding the balance in your life.

Be sure your informational highway (your nervous system) is in balance as well. A curve in your communication system may make your journey to health much more treacherous. Adding daily exercise or yoga will tune that fine engine of yours. Once you begin some lifestyle changes and address some of your health issues, your energy level will begin to return. Don't be afraid to try to find the true answers to your health conditions. Magic pills will not cure the problem; they only mask the symptoms.

Chapter 7
Who Is Sleeping Beautifully?

Oh to be sleeping beauty for just one night! How many days or months has it been since you slept all night, got up on your own and felt like a new woman? You would think that if you are physically in adrenal exhaustion then you could sleep, right? Actually, it can be just the opposite.

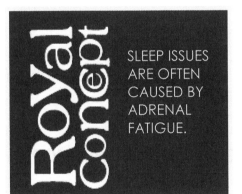

SLEEP ISSUES ARE OFTEN CAUSED BY ADRENAL FATIGUE.

You may not be aware that difficulty sleeping is one of the most common symptoms of a woman who has too much stress and an incomplete "Circle of Health."

Remember, when one organ or gland is not functioning properly, others have to try and act as a back-up. After a while, your body begins to shut down if it can't get what it needs. Your body will try very hard to naturally heal itself. The only way you have a chance to heal yourself is to sleep. If your sleep pattern is off, you cannot maintain health.

If cortisol levels are too high at night, rather than getting the rest and recovery necessary to maintain optimal physical repair and psychic regeneration, your body will be in a catabolic state (high nighttime cortisol levels inhibit the release of growth hormone necessary to repair and rebuild body tissues).

High cortisol will also have a negative effect on brain function, memory, learning and mood. This is especially true if this condition is ongoing (chronic in nature). This state can literally make you think you are going crazy, when really your adrenals are just exhausted.

Are you dreaming or are you living the fairytale? Do you sleep like you have been put under a spell or do you feel fantastic and rested when you wake up? Do you awaken ready to go and face the world? Or are you one of many who can't even remember the last night you experienced a sound, full night of sleep?

A good night's sleep is often the best way to help you cope with stress, solve problems, or recover from illness. Let's have some fun now that we know so much about sleep.

WHICH FAIRYTALE DESCRIBES YOUR SLEEPING?

Sleeping Beauty enjoys 8 to 10 hours of sound, uninterrupted sleep each night, and sleeps marvelously, almost as if a spell has been placed on her. She experiences ideal, deep, and restful sleep, while dreaming about wonderful moments to come. She wakes up feeling refreshed and ready for the beautiful day ahead.

Sleeping Beauty has a complete "Circle of Health." Her body heals and rebuilds itself as she sleeps. She maintains good health by practicing nutritional habits and moderate daily exercise.

A balanced lifestyle will help Sleeping Beauty achieve more from life with prince charming and decrease the effects of natural aging. She will be rested and well-prepared for the stress that comes unexpectedly from wicked birthday crashers and other fiendish turn-of-events!

The Princess and the Pea sleeps very lightly. Any little noise awakens her. A bird outside...the humming of the AC...whispering in the hallway...her eyes are opened, guaranteed. She can't get comfortable, feels that pea underneath her mattress, and every ache, pain, and stress associated with it. She can't seem to get into a deeper sleep pattern. She's at her wit's end.

The Princess and the Pea has symptoms of adrenal fatigue from an over-stressed life. For example, a new mother or a caretaker of an elderly or sick family member can have some of these same issues. Adrenal glands will be exhausted from the stress of daily activities, and sex hormones (estrogen and/or progesterone) are usually deficient in some manner. This makes sense since the adrenal glands, which provide our stress hormones, cannot back them up. Her "Circle of Health" has a couple of missing pieces that need to be corrected for the circle to function and for her health to return. She may be making poor nutritional choices and getting little to no exercise to help combat stress.

This princess would benefit from lifestyle changes, along with nutritional supplementation such as B & C vitamins and minerals. Testing for hormone levels of estrogen, progesterone, testosterone, cortisol and DHEA would identify deficiencies, and supplementation with bio-identical hormones can replenish the deficiencies. With the right supplements, she could return to a life of peaceful slumber with her prince in a short period of time.

Cinderella before the ball is so excited she can hardly stand it. She is very anxious about all the details, keeping her mind so busy and full of thoughts. She may not want to fall asleep because of all the excitement. She may fall asleep for a couple of hours, and then at the stroke of midnight awaken and spend the rest of the night tossing and turning while thinking ... thinking ... thinking about all the details dancing around in her head.

Cinderella is experiencing adrenal fatigue because of extended periods of anxiety and excitement about her busy life. This causes her sleep to be restless and dissatisfying. Her body and mind need sleep to heal and to process thoughts properly. She worries about the details that she might be forgetting and is desperate for the sleep that she cannot attain. Her "Circle of Health" needs attention in key areas of imbalance.

Lifestyle changes such as making her bedtime routine more relaxing, foregoing the alcoholic nightcap and replacing it with a relaxing bath, creating a quiet, darkened environment and removing distractions such a television could all be beneficial. Hormone levels such as estrogen and progesterone should be tested, along with neurotransmitter levels such as dopamine, epinephrine and serotonin. Any deficiencies should be replaced along with good nutritional support, B vitamins and minerals. Some herbal relaxants like valerian root may help Cinderella feel drowsy. Having energy to go shopping for those glass slippers is right around the corner with proper testing and supplements, along with a few lifestyle changes.

Snow White and the poisoned apple is knocked out with medication because she has no other option. She is dependent on a sleep aid to fall asleep. She sleeps for 8-10 hours in what appears to be deep sleep, but awakens feeling tired, unmotivated towards the day. She has no extra energy to take care of herself, much less her hardworking family and friends.

Snow White may be suffering from adrenal fatigue (too much stress), hormonal deficiencies (menopause), neurotransmitter imbalance, poor nutrition, and toxicities. There are numerous possibilities of what might be her underlying cause of insomnia.

Appropriate testing is a must to find the exact answer of what will bring Snow White back to reality. More than likely she has a combination of hormone deficiencies intensified by adrenal gland exhaustion. Her endocrine system is the first place to look for testing, correction and support.

Snow White can barely get through life because she has no circadian rhythm or natural sleep pattern left. She has completely altered her body's ability to achieve rest. She must make a huge lifestyle change to slowly get off her medications that are inhibiting her natural sleep patterns and must strive to find the reason she is not sleeping on her own. This could be stress, hormone deficiencies, nutritional or toxicity issues. She must work towards finding out what her real issues are regarding her "Circle of Health."

She is attacking her symptom of sleep disturbance with sleep aids, but not finding out the true cause of her problems. Consider an alternative sleep aid like melatonin. It may help reach the deeper layers of sleep without feeling drowsy. Achieving balance both mentally and physically will help restore Snow White to feeling like singing "High Ho," and going off to work once again.

In order to get a good night's sleep, you need to look into your overall health and wellness. There is an underlying dysfunction that is contributing to your disrupted circadian rhythm. Sleepless nights can be a nightmare. If you dig deeper into your health, you can regain the life of your dreams.

SLEEP ON IT!

The phrase "I'll sleep on it 'til morning" has real meaning. You need rest for your brain to recharge for the next day's stresses. Have you ever just finished final exams or a huge project at work, and then, bam—you come down with a terrible cold? That's no accident! Sleep is essential to the immune system. Without adequate sleep, the immune system begins to weaken, and the body becomes more vulnerable to infection and disease.

Sleep is also a time of rest and repair to neurons. Neurons are the freeways of the nervous system that carry out both voluntary commands, like moving your arm, and involuntary commands, like breathing and digestive processes. Many of the hormones or substances that are produced to trigger or regulate particular body functions are timed to release during sleep or right before sleep. Growth hormones, for example, are released during sleep. These hormones are vital not only to growing children, but also to adults for restorative processes like muscle repair.

SHEDDING SOME LIGHT ON SLEEP

Melatonin is the hormone produced by the pineal gland which helps with our sleep cycles and is intimately linked to light. The pineal gland responds to the amount of light taken in by the eye, which helps to determine the circadian rhythm. We start off our mornings with high Cortisol levels and low melatonin levels. This allows us to start the day feeling fresh and ready for the daily stressors.

> **Melatonin is a hormone responsible for helping our sleep cycle.**

You use up approximately half of your cortisol by noon. By afternoon another half is gone, so by nighttime your body must produce melatonin to help you go to sleep. Normally, melatonin levels begin to rise in the mid to late evening, and remain high for most of the night, dropping in the early morning hours.

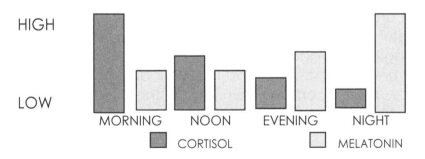

By now you are beginning to see how there really is a dance-like rhythm of cortisol and melatonin hormones swirling around the dance floor of your life. If one hormone gets out of step, it affects you. You can't sleep!

THE RHYTHM OF SLEEP

Your body has a natural rhythm for sleep. We all have an internal circadian clock that provides cues for when it's time to sleep and time to wake. This clock is sensitive to light and time of day, which is why having a good bedtime routine and a quiet, dark place to sleep, is so important.

At the same time, a chemical messenger called adenosine builds up during the day as our bodies are busy using energy. The more adenosine builds up in the brain, the sleepier you will feel. Adenosine combined with the circadian clock sends a powerful message of sleepiness to your body.

A SECOND WIND

Have you ever experienced a second wind late at night while working on a project and stayed up even later than anticipated? This happens often you experience a stressful and busy work career. That was your cortisol kicking back in again before the morning influx because your body was stressed and told your adrenal glands to make more cortisol. Remember the normal table above? This is what the second wind looks like!

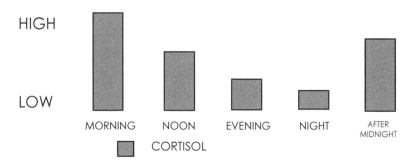

SLEEP DISORDERS

There are four main categories of Sleep Disorders, which affect your ability to fall asleep: lifestyle, health complications, medication side effects and clinical disorders.

Lifestyle
The main lifestyle concerns when dealing with sleep disorders are the late night use of caffeine or alcohol. Caffeine is a stimulant, and if you drink it in the evening, it may make it hard to fall asleep. Alcohol is a depressant; so many people think it will help them sleep. It might help you fall asleep, but it usually acts as a stimulant, waking you up throughout the night. Your diet at night and throughout the whole day can contribute to your restless nights.

Working the late night shift might put more money in your pocket, but at what cost? Your natural body's circadian rhythm will be greatly affected by this unnatural shift of sleep pattern. Working in different time zones traveling back and forth? Jet lag also confuses your natural rhythm.

Health Complications
Health complications are always a potential issue for sleep disorders. Pregnancy can keep you from getting comfortable, and you're probably getting up to go potty 5 times a night! If you are injured physically, this can cause sleeping challenges.

Sleep apnea and is affecting more people by the minute. You may think you just suffer from snoring when in actuality it is sleep apnea. A sleep study might be needed to properly diagnosis the issue. Sleep apnea is a condition where you actually stop breathing during sleep and jerk and gasp for breath. It is extremely hard on your heart and allows you to get very little restful and healing sleep. It is hard to get sound sleep while dealing with these types of health complications.

Medication Side Effects

Many medications, both prescription and over the counter, can cause the side effect of insomnia. Many people taking medicines for a particular ailment may attribute their sleep issues to the problem instead of the cure. Some antidepressants can cause the onset of REM Sleep Disorder. People have been known to physically act out their dreams while fully asleep.

Antihistamines can cause drowsiness during the day, and result in disrupted sleep patterns at night. Decongestants taken too close to bedtime have the ability to excite and increase alertness, making it very tough to fall asleep.

Asthma medications increase breath intake but decrease time asleep and the soundness of that sleep. Most weight loss medications have a diuretic or stimulant like caffeine as their main ingredient. Their goal is to rev up the body's metabolism.

A diuretic will make you need to go to the bathroom to urinate, while the stimulant will overexcite the mind and make it difficult to fall asleep.

Ironically, sleep medications can often exacerbate the exact problem they are designed to help. Sleep aids should be used only for a short period of time or they will override the body's natural sleep mechanism, making the body forget how to lull itself to sleep without assistance.

Clinical Disorders

Clinical Disorders can include asthmatics that have difficulty breathing, substance abusers, and depressed or highly stressed individuals. You may need to stop watching your 401-K, or try to quit obsessing about the stock market or worrying about potential layoffs. These things may literally be keeping you awake at night.

Concern about the current state of the economy is taking its toll on our sleep habits. According to a survey by the Washington-based National Sleep Foundation, one third of Americans are losing sleep over the state of the economy. The number of patients seeking treatment for insomnia is up 10 percent in the past year.

HOW MUCH SLEEP DO YOU REALLY NEED?

The need for sleep depends on various factors, one of which is age. Infants usually require about 16-18 hours of sleep per day, while teenagers need about 9 hours per day on average. Most adults need about 7-8 hours of sleep per day, but the amount of sleep a person needs depends on the individual.

Sleep Requirements:	
Infants	16 - 18 hours / day
Teenagers	9 hours / day
Adults	7 - 8 hours / day

DEEP SLEEP IS WHAT YOU SEEK

Now that we understand what might be the cause of your problem sleeping, let's review what makes up a good night's sleep. There are two main types of sleep. REM (Rapid Eye Movement) sleep is when you do your most active dreaming.

Your eyes actually move back and forth during this stage, which is why it is called REM sleep. Non-REM (NREM) sleep consists of four stages of deeper and deeper sleep. Each sleep stage is important for overall quality sleep, but deep sleep and REM sleep are especially vital.

SWEET DREAMS

REM sleep, or dream sleep, is essential to our minds for processing and consolidating emotions, memories and stress. It is also thought to be vital to learning, stimulating the brain regions used in learning and developing new skills. Most of dreaming occurs during REM sleep.

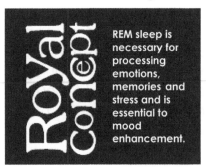

REM sleep is necessary for processing emotions, memories and stress and is essential to mood enhancement.

Studies have shown that better REM sleep helps boost your mood during the day. This is referred to as REM sleep, when the body is trying to rebuild tissues, fight infections and inflammation and in general just recover.

HOW CAN YOU GET MORE REM SLEEP?

One simple way is to try to sleep a little more in the morning. As your sleep cycles through the night, it starts with longer periods of deep sleep. By the morning, the

REM sleep stage is longer. Try sleeping an extra 30 minutes to one hour and see if your mood improves. If your body is deprived of deep sleep, it will try to make that up first—at the expense of REM sleep.

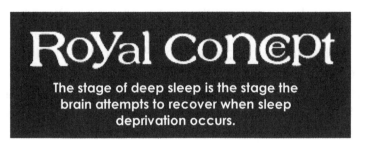

Royal Conept

The stage of deep sleep is the stage the brain attempts to recover when sleep deprivation occurs.

DEEP SLEEP IS VITAL

Each stage of sleep offers benefits to the sleeper. However, deep sleep is perhaps the most vital stage. What might disrupt deep sleep? If you are caring for someone around the clock, whether a small infant or an elderly relative with a serious illness, you might need to attend to them suddenly in the middle of the night.

Loud noises outside or inside the home might wake you. If you work the night shift, sleeping during the day may be difficult, due to light and excess noise during the day. Substances like alcohol and nicotine also disrupt deep sleep. You must maximize your deep sleep.

Make sure your sleep environment is as comfortable as possible and try to minimize outside noises. If you are being awakened as a caregiver, make sure that you get some uninterrupted sleep, especially if you have had some unusually disruptive nights. Don't be afraid to ask for help. Remember, you are a queen.

NIGHT, NIGHT SLEEP TIGHT

Too little sleep may cause impaired memory and thought processes, depression, and a decrease in your immune response. Now you know why sleep is so important to your health and well being. You have to make it a priority in your life to get a good sleep routine and a rhythm in place nightly. For short periods of time, a sleep aid may be necessary; but use them with caution. Remember, sleep aids are habit forming. Lifestyle and behavioral changes are the best action to take.

HERE ARE SOME SUGGESTIONS TO GET A GOOD NIGHT'S SLEEP

- A good night's sleep starts during the day by practicing good "sleep hygiene." Exercise and eating balanced meals are important.

- Coffee and other caffeine products—even chocolate—should not be consumed after dinner so that the caffeine has time to dissipate.

- In the evening, a warm shower or bath can serve as a way to lull the body to relax.

- The bedroom should be used for its original purposes—sleep and sex—and that's all. Turn off the TV, banish the computer to another room, draw the shades or pull the curtains. Turn the clock around or cover its bright light. Retrain your pet to sleep in his own space rather than yours.

- During the hour or two before bed, reprogram your brain to formally set aside daily worries. Do not pay bills right before bed.

- A cocktail or glass of wine is a false sleep aid. Alcohol can cause a stimulant effect that kicks in and wakes you up after a few hours. Switch to chamomile tea or warm milk.

- Lower the thermostat in the bedroom or crack a window open slightly. It's easier for the body to sleep in a cool space than a stuffy, over-heated one.

- Listen to your iPod and favorite mellow music to relax.

- Finally, pick up something easy to read.

CUT 2 THE CHASE:

The "Circle of Health" philosophy strongly emphasizes that you must go to sleep and get some rest in order to address your stress. It is the only way your body can repair itself. You may need a sleep aid while you are being tested to find out the true deficiencies in your system, or maybe you just need to supplement melatonin until you get balanced.

Remember, staying on sleep medications or supplements for too long will shut down your pineal glands from producing or manufacturing your own melatonin and the feedback loop will be broken; thus, your circadian rhythm will no longer be able to dance.

Test to rule out sleep apnea if you are your partner is concerned about excessive snoring. The continual strain on your heart could be too much eventually.

Once your "Circle of Health" returns to a healthier, better well-rounded circle, you should notice sleeping becomes subconscious like it should be. Sleep tight, and don't let the bed bugs bite!

Chapter 8
Relevant Testing and Solutions

BACK TO SCHOOL

Riiiiiinnnnnnnggggg! Get up!

It's time for school. It's time for health education 101. You have to take control of your own health. In order to do your best, you are going to have to do your homework. Seeking out the best health care professional to help you get your "Circle of Health" put back in place is essential, but you will also need a good textbook.

We hope you find this chapter an excellent reference and guide to the material you need to know in order to get tested properly.

Think of relevant testing as if you are taking a test and getting a grade. The proper testing will show you a thorough view of your current health. Invest in yourself; you are worth it!

BACK TO THE BASICS

It's quiz time! What are the four key components of the "Circle of Health"? Can you name them? Hormones, Nutrition, Purification, and Neurons.

Great job! When you are experiencing health issues just go back and review the basics. Decide which crown jewel has got trouble.

Remember, it may not be just one. By at least acknowledging the possibilities of the core underlying condition of your symptoms, you have already made a passing grade.

Breaking this chapter of testing and solutions into the four main crown jewels is how we are going to approach this broad topic.

We can only briefly hit the major topics and tests; we feel these are most important with the oral systemic link, but there are many other tests that can guide you to your best treatment. These just reveal some great information quickly and easily.

HORMONES

When people hear the word hormones, their natural tendency is to think of female sex hormones like estrogen and the crazy ups and downs that many woman experience through puberty, PMS, pregnancy, or menopause.

But remember: the sex organs are not the only organs that use hormones to regulate systems in the body. The thyroid and adrenal glands control vital bodily systems.

To clarify, a hormone is simply a chemical released by a cell in one part of the body that sends out messages that affect cells in other parts of the body.

ADRENAL TESTING

Don't forget: the main goal of this book has been to help you uncover the huge contribution the adrenal glands make to a stressful life, so that you can address the stress.

So how do you discover if you have adrenal exhaustion or fatigue? Cortisol and DHEA can be tested via blood or saliva: let's take a look at both.

Saliva testing for hormones is a preferred method for testing cortisol and DHEA (as well as estrogen, testosterone, and progesterone) because it allows your practitioner to see what is bio-available (free floating) and therefore usable by your tissues.

Blood tests measure the levels of hormones that are physically attached to the red blood cells, but not what is free floating and in a more usable or available state.

Optimal adrenal function exists when the ratio of cortisol to DHEA is in proper balance. This is why measuring this ratio is the best way to evaluate adrenal function and determine the effect stress is having on your overall health.

STAGE I ADRENAL FATIGUE	HIGH CORTISOL / HIGH DHEA
STAGE II ADRENAL FATIGUE	NORMAL CORTISOL / LOW DHEA
STAGE III ADRENAL FATIGUE	LOW CORTISOL / LOW DHEA

If cortisol and DHEA are elevated, your adrenals are responding to stress, but they are still fairly healthy (STAGE I ADRENAL FATIGUE).

If cortisol is normal and DHEA is low, your adrenals are still responding to stress, but they are getting fatigued (STAGE II).

If your cortisol and DHEA are both low, then the adrenals are really starting to wane in production (STAGE III).

When this happens, you lose your ability to regulate bodily functions and are on the road to further hormone, immune, and metabolic breakdown. Maintaining physiological balance is an important aspect of vibrant health, and nowhere is this more evident than when it comes to cortisol. The production of too much cortisol can literally burn up your body, and insufficient cortisol production causes your body's internal machinery to malfunction, especially at the cellular level.

Let's talk about supporting the adrenal hormones. If you discover that you are in Stage II or III of adrenal fatigue, then your protocol could include supplementing cortisol, DHEA and pregnenolone. Supplementing adrenal hormones allows you to immediately feel better while allowing your adrenals to heal.

What is pregnenolone? We thought you would never ask.

Pregnenolone is the first hormone the adrenals produce, and it has the choice of becoming cortisol for stress or DHEA for backup to the sex hormones—testosterone and estrogen.

Pregnenolone "shifts" to the production of cortisol when your body is in a constant stress response. Your body is more concerned about managing your stress response than backing up your sex hormones. Under times of extreme stress, reproduction of sex hormones is put on the back burner.

So that is why if your adrenals are exhausted, it is recommended to supplement pregnenolone. *It is what you need initially to combat stress.*

SEX HORMONES

By the time most of you have symptoms of adrenal fatigue, you are in your mid to late 30's. You experience adrenal fatigue in this age range because of your busy lifestyle. Going hand-in-hand with this, your sex hormones also begin to naturally decline as your age increases.

Let's look at men first. As men age, their testosterone and progesterone levels decrease and their estrogen levels become more prominent. Because of this, we test sex hormones in men in addition to the adrenals through their saliva. In this case, saliva testing is the preferred method over blood testing. Saliva results will show sex hormones that are more available directly to the tissues, while blood tests will only report hormones that are attached to red blood cells.

The concern for men is to increase their testosterone and progesterone in order to counteract the estrogenic effects that older men have to deal with, such as prostate problems and breast cancer. An increase in testosterone will help give back energy, drive, ambition, libido, etc. Removing stress will only help the production of sex hormones, because the adrenals are also the backup system to the testicles. Supplementing hormones will decrease the stress on the adrenals since they are no longer being relied on for hormone production.

When testing for sex hormones in women, a saliva test is also preferred. For the same reason that was mentioned in the male testing scenario, the bio-availability information received from a saliva test will give much more information than a blood test. Since the adrenals back up the woman's sex glands or ovaries, the more we can elevate the sex hormones (estrogen, progesterone, and testosterone) the more we can allow the adrenal glands a chance to rest and recover.

Pre-menopause

Pre-menopausal women are typically deficient in progesterone because they are ovulating less frequently. It is very important that you supplement with a bio-identical progesterone that matches your body, rather than a synthetic hormone. To avoid nasty side effects, it is to go with hormones that molecularly are most similar to your natural hormone makeup.

Menopause

Menopausal women are deficient in estrogen and progesterone. Again, it is important that you supplement with both bio-identical estrogen and progesterone that matches your body rather than with synthetic hormones. Balance is the key. When in menopause, you must produce a mimicked effect of the natural cycle you used to have. Woman will have a surge of estrogen in mid-month, followed by a surge of progesterone. You experience the surge of estrogen in order to help your body's progesterone receptors receive progesterone.   You will have a surge of progesterone to help your body's estrogen receptors receive estrogen at the beginning of your next cycle.

The natural cycle of a woman protects her bone, mental, and physical overall health. Without these protective processes continuing to occur, your aging process will accelerate.

Andropause

For men age 45-60, testosterone depletes about one percent a year as they age. Bio-identical testosterone and progesterone are very important for the health of the prostate.

THYROID TESTING

If you have been experiencing chronic stress, then your thyroid needs to be tested. The adrenals help back up the thyroid, which helps determine your metabolic rate. If you continually try to lose weight and never see a change, run a complete test on your thyroid to check your metabolism. The thyroid needs to be working optimally to remove the stress and strain from the adrenal glands. The thyroid must be tested via blood.

You should have a four to seven panel comprehensive thyroid test, included in these are:

TSH-Thyroid Stimulating Hormone

T3-Triiodothyronine
T4-Thyroxine
Reverse T3
T3 uptake
T7 calculated
Thyroid antibodies

Here in a nutshell is the main message about testing the thyroid: be sure to get a full vision of thyroid activity by a more complete panel or test.

The standard Thyroid test seems to be TSH, or thyroid stimulating hormone, but that test alone does not reveal the entire picture. It does not even test the thyroid itself. It tests the feedback from the pituitary. The pituitary gland produces TSH, not the thyroid.

Usually your thyroid is only tested by looking at a level of TSH, which is a messenger hormone produced by the pituitary gland. TSH's function is to tell your thyroid to produce more T3 and T4. This measurement could be faulty if your pituitary is not functioning properly or if the feedback mechanism from your thyroid is off in some way. We suggest knowing exactly what your thyroid gland is doing.

The function of your thyroid can be very confusing. The biggest debate we have is when to use medications and whether to use Synthroid or Armour.

T3, Triiodothyronine, functions as the more active thyroid hormone; whereas T4, Triiodothyronine, is more of the storage form. Synthroid is an example of T4 hormone and Armour is a combination of T3 and T4, giving you active forms of both hormones.

If you have trouble converting T4 (the storage form) into the more active T3, you could have a high level of T4 and a low level of TSH (meaning your test results look fine), but you would still feel awful. This is exactly why only the full panel of thyroid testing will reveal the exact issues you may or may not be having. We are huge fans of Armour Thyroid, which is bio-identical T3 and T4 hormones that is very effective. Optimizing your thyroid will help relieve the adrenals and allow them to recover from fatigue.

Remember, your endocrine system is a closed system, and one or two glands being out of balance will fatigue your adrenals. That is why we suggest you test your sex hormones, adrenals, and thyroid together most of the time.

NUTRITION

GLUCOSE/PANCREAS TESTING
Many of us have gotten use to the idea of a supersized world. We loved it when we felt like we were getting more for our money. Believe you me: we were getting more—more fat, more calories, more weight, and more unhealthiness.

Stop now and look at how much you eat versus how much you really need to give yourself good and healthy nutrition. You will be surprised! If you are overweight, have any family history of diabetes, or experience the highs and lows of blood sugar, then please dedicate yourself immediately to taking a first step toward helping your over all wellness. Move towards testing and making a change in your eating habits.

Your glucose level and pancreatic function is critical to the health of the adrenal glands. Your adrenals back up your pancreas and the balancing of blood sugar. Testing your fasting blood glucose will reveal if you are having issues with your blood sugar. Hemoglobin A1C will test pancreatic function. If your glucose or Hemoglobin A1C test levels are high, a solution could be to place you on a low glycemic diet in order to get your weight down. You could possibly be prescribed some medications like Glucophage or Metformin in order to balance your blood sugar until your weight is under control.

Diabetes is a chronic inflammatory disease, and for many people can easily be controlled by weight loss and a healthier nutritional lifestyle. If you only believed how much better you would feel, you wouldn't waste another day putting this off. It is a life changer! You are so worth it!

FOOD SENSITIVITY

Food sensitivities can cause inflammation of your small intestine, which causes an increased permeability or "leaky gut." This in turn allows allergens, yeast, and parasites into your bloodstream, which puts your immune system on alert. Once this happens, your body starts to try to fight the inflammation systemically. Arthritis and other inflammatory diseases have been linked to food sensitivities for this reason.

Food sensitivities are tested via a blood test for IgG sensitivity to foods. This is different from IgE reactions which are food allergies. With IgG sensitivities, there is a 48 to 72 hour delayed response which can show up as abdominal pain, headaches, skin irritations, etc. IgE is a blood test or skin scratch test which shows an immediate response. We find that by testing your food sensitivities (IgG), more is revealed clinically that might easily go unnoticed. Things you ate two days ago that you have no memory of eating could be wreaking havoc with your system. That's where the blood test comes in handy; it can identify the exact foods causing the issue. Gluten seems to be a very common food sensitivity in our community right now.

A special diet is developed for the removal of specific foods for 21 days; this allows your body to recover from sensitivities. Once your small intestine has had time to heal, the foods can slowly be reintroduced back into your diet on a rotational basis--typically a four day rotation diet. This rotational diet keeps you from getting sensitized to that food again. You might add a probiotic to your daily regimen. A probiotic will replenish the healthy flora in your digestive system. We are all exposed to things like E. coli and staphylococcus, and if you have taken antibiotics long term, your digestive system may have been robbed of its healthy flora. Antibiotics kill both the good and the bad bacteria, so a probiotic is a good counter measure to help replenish the healthy natural flora.

Once again, food sensitivities or an imbalance in our micro-flora places more stress on our adrenal glands. In response the adrenals must produce Cortisol, your body's natural response to inflammation.

NUTRITIONAL DEFICIENCIES: ALPHABET SOUP

Let's talk about the attributes of vitamins and minerals and the importance of adding them to your daily regimen.

If your food sources are organic, free of pesticides, and you eat a diet heavily weighted in vegetables and fruit, you may not need to worry about supplementing; however, if this is not the case, then you may want to see what you're missing. Consider the following list as your recipe for alphabet soup...

Vitamin A	Healthy vision, immunity, bone metabolism
Vitamin Bs	Energy production, reduces inflammation, nerve health
Vitamin C	Antioxidant, immunity, counteracts stress
Calcium	Bone and teeth health, muscle contraction
Copper	Red blood cells, collagen, immunity
Vitamin D3	Fights cancer, bone health, reduces inflammation
Vitamin E	Antioxidant, blood thinner
Folic Acid	Manufactures red blood cells
Flavinoids (Vitamin P)	Improves absorption of Vitamin C
Glutathione	Antioxidant, immunity
Vitamin H (Biotin)	Growth and development, hair, nails
Iodine	Required for thyroid hormones
Iron	Oxygenation, metabolizing B vitamins
Vitamin K	Blood clotting
Magnesium	Nerves, muscle contraction, lower high blood pressure, immunity
Manganese	Cartilage and bone
Niacin	DNA repair, production of adrenal hormones, reduces cholesterol
Omega 3 Essential Fatty Acids	Reduces inflammation, depression
Potassium	Lowers blood pressure, electrolyte, muscle contraction
Riboflavin	Energy metabolism
Selenium	Prevents cancer, cardiovascular disease, anti-aging
Thiamine	Breaks down sugar in the diet
Zinc	Needed for every cell in body, immunity, wound healing, taste & smell

A simple blood test can reveal any essential vitamins or nutrients your body desperately needs to function properly.

PH BALANCE

To sustain the body of a royal queen, there is another hierarchy to consider—the priorities for survival. Second only to breathing and a heartbeat, the most important metabolic function is maintaining a specific pH.

The term pH stands for potential hydrogen or the amount of hydrogen ions in a solution. The more ions in a solution, the higher the acidity level; and the fewer ions, the more alkaline or basic is in the solution. pH is measured on a scale from zero to fourteen, with seven being neutral or mid-range.

Many things can influence the pH balance of a person: stress, poor nutritional choices, medications, etc. Any drop in pH, no matter how slight, is the beginning of a disease state and affects when and how we age. All other organs and fluids will fluctuate in their range in order to keep the blood at a strict pH between 7.35 and 7.45. This process is called homeostasis.

You can easily monitor your pH with simple testing strips which can be purchased at your local pharmacy.

Testing saliva is the easiest way to gauge the body's pH. To test saliva: Wait two hours after eating. Spit into a spoon. Dip the strip. Read immediately. Use the color chart included. An optimal reading is 7.5. This indicates a very slightly alkaline body.

Urine is more acidic than saliva. To test urine: Test a urine sample first thing in the morning. Fill a small cup with urine, and dip a strip into the cup. Read immediately. An optimal reading is about 6.5.

In the mouth, your saliva could have an increased pH

level if you suffer from acidic reflux, indigestion, or gird. The stomach pH is much higher in acidity due to the need for hydrochloric acid to begin the digestion of food.

If your mouth experiences a sustained higher level of acidity, you could suffer from an increase of cavities, dental or periodontal infections. Combine this issue with a dry mouth and a perfect storm will arise and create many dental, and sinus related problems.

Preventive and proactive measures need to be made on people with history of stomach or acid issues, and don't forget pregnancies. Many women suffer from acid reflux and vomiting for prolonged period of times.

A small amount may not affect your teeth, but multiple months and multiple pregnancies will certainly take a toll on your teeth if you are not proactive. It is important to keep that royal blood line growing, but not at the expense of losing the queen's beautiful smile.

The simplest way to balance out a pH balance is through your diet. It is recommended to eat 75% of alkaline foods, but the typical American diet consists of an 85% acid food source. Increase your raw vegetables and fresh fruit and cut back on caffeinated soda drinks.

PURIFICATION

Cardiovascular Testing
Cardiovascular Testing is more important than you might ever imagine. Why wait till you are in the midst of a cardio event before you consider your heart health. Many people love that big heart you have and want

you around to share the joys of life for years to come with them. If you don't care about yourself, then maybe considering that others do will be enough of a reason to stop and move forward with testing your LOVE status – your heart!

Listen carefully to this. If you have ANY family history of heart disease, it may be a larger positive risk factor for you than smoking! What we mean by this is you could smoke a pack a day and never suffer from a cardiac event if your family genes do not predestine you to cardiac disease. Unbelievable, I know.

So here are three easy tests to look into as soon as possible.

DNA Saliva Testing

DNA saliva testing is now available through your dentist to help diagnose bacteria in your mouth that can be in your entire blood stream, contributing to the plaque buildup in your arteries and leading to cardiovascular disease. By taking a small saliva sample, you can identify what type and how much of bad pathogens are present in your system. This correlates to the risk factor you have for cardiovascular disease, diabetes, stroke, and some forms of cancer.

The oral-systemic link now has compelling evidence of the correlation between the chronic inflammatory destruction of many of these disease processes. If someone has been diagnosed with periodontal disease or cardiac disease, then he or she must aggressively treat both health issues because of their close correlation of the exact same pathogen or bad bacterial cause.

The saliva test results will identify exactly which pathogens are present, and a specific antibiotic regimen can be given to eradicate the bacteria—not only from your mouth, but also throughout your entire blood stream. You may also need to take a much more aggressive approach to cleaning your teeth; perhaps localized treatment with antibiotics, and antimicrobial mouthwashes are needed for the first wave of attack. You may also need to increase your cleaning to once every three months rather than six months to allow professionals to disrupt the biofilm around your teeth and to keep the areas from bleeding. Retesting at six weeks post treatment will confirm success of the removal of the pathogens.

With the presence of bleeding, you have a direct wound allowing bacteria into your entire blood stream. How long would you leave a bleeding open wound stay on your hand? Would it take you even a day before you went and got stitches? So why is it ok that your gums bleed when you brush or floss? It is not ok!

If you also have a family history of heart disease, strokes, or diabetes, then go to your dentist soon armed with this new technology and ask for the testing called MyPerioPath Test form Oral DNA labs. It could be life changing for you.

You will also want your dentist to run the My Perio PST Test. This test only has to be run once. It is basically a saliva test that is a genetic marker for inflammation. About 30% of Caucasians will be positive. A positive test result would reveal that you are more likely to respond to any injury or illness with inflammation, meaning you are at a higher risk for diabetes, heart disease, stroke, cancers, periodontal disease, allergies, arthritis, autoimmune disease, etc.

With news like that, many people would be scared of the result. I say don't be scared: be thrilled that you know now. Get with the program and realize you must focus that much harder on changing your life to a healthier one. You are genetically more predisposed to the underlying health issues. You need to make a BIG focused effort on change and live a more preventive life. And you just may find the hidden secret to some of your previous health concerns.

CIMT

It is the most non-invasive way as a first screening for cardiovascular disease. CIMT stands for Carotid Intima-Media Thickness and is a painless diagnostic ultrasound of the carotids in your neck. It measures the soft plaque accumulation levels within the walls of your arteries. The presence of significant soft plaque could be vulnerable to rupture and create a cardiac event. So, early detection and intervention is critical for both men and women.

HPV Oral Cancer Testing

Through a simple non invasive saliva test, you can find answers to your current risk factors for HPV induced oral cancers. If you have had a history of HPV exposure, then you should consider this test. Even though there are many strains of the HPV virus, two in particular are now both present in sexual transmission and the root cause of oral cancer.

For years the high risk patient for oral cancer was a white male 50 years or older that had long term history of tobacco use. Now our population is changing unexpectedly due to HPV. We now are seeing oral cancer increase in woman ages 30 to 60 with no history of smoking at all or tobacco use of any kind.

In the future, we will see more tests examining the DNA in saliva that determine the risks a person has for cancer. Early prevention and detection is an easy way to keep us healthy.

Heavy Metal Testing
Geographically there are some areas that have higher risks for heavy metal toxins. Identifying lead, mercury, and other heavy metals might be important in your line of work or due to environmental factors. Heavy metal toxins of all kinds can be tested easily through hair samples or via blood. Detoxification regimens can be done to help remove and release the unwanted levels.

NERVOUS

Chiropractor Evaluation
A clear message sent and a clear message received are so important in life with your relationships, co-workers, and your body parts. Without proper communication your foundation of relationships, work, or health will crumple. A chiropractic evaluation may need to be done to make sure your alignment is appropriate. An active childhood or trauma in the past could have moved things out of their ideal position. As you had youth on your side it might have been unnoticed. But as you age this underlying curve in your highway may begin to take you off track.

TMJ pain, fibromyalgia, chronic pain and trauma are good examples of how your body can be damaged so your body parts can no longer send and receive a clear message. Maybe your trauma is way past the simple help of a chiropractor due to down or broken pieces of your skeletal and muscular system. Then just be sure you understand what the underlying health condition may be contributing to. Like a phone dropping a cal or static on the line, it can be difficult to hear and frustration begins. Body parts and organs may not be able to send out the messages they need for health or for help. Dig down to the source of your problem.

Let's share an example. A woman comes to her dental appointment almost six months overdue and has been a great patient for many years. She has always been upbeat and energetic.

Now she seems overweight and lethargic, her oral health is poor, and she has come in with devastating migraines that she can no longer cope with. After discussing her previous health changes over the last six months, the underlying cause of her health deterioration is revealing itself.

She fell this winter and severely broke her knee and elbow on the ice. She has been under surgery four times to correct the issues, which still seem to be causing her trouble. She can't sleep, she is depressed, she can't eat because her jaw hurts, and she has no energy or motivation to take care of herself anymore.

Let's go to the "Circle of Health" and identify a few of her underlying health conditions.

Hormones: adrenal exhaustion due to recent surgeries and trying to heal from trauma, increases symptoms of her pre-menopause because the adrenals are no longer able to back up sex hormones. Metabolism has decreased, and she put on weight from having no back up to her thyroid and her recent lack of exercise.

Nutrition: She verges on diabetes now with her weight gain, lack of exercise and issues with her high and low blood sugars. Even though she desperately craves sugar and sweets all the time, she can't eat because it hurts her jaw. Her stomach stays upset all the time now and she suffers from acid reflux terribly.

Purification: Her periodontal and oral health is in bad shape now due to poor nutrition and hygiene, while her clenching and grinding is at an all time high even though she feels like her teeth do not touch properly anymore. She now is concerned she might be having heart issues.

Neurons: Her aches and pains are at an all time high while her migraines are debilitating and increasing in number monthly.

Believe it or not all these things began with one simple accident on ice. It just began a snowball effect on her health. Each problem leads to an underlying core issue that began to weave itself intricately through the "Circle of Health". She can get back on track, but she needs to take control of her own health again and make some very proactive approaches to get healthy again.

Adjustment can help realign hips, back, neck, and TMJ joints from trauma or surgeries. This realignment can increase the communication of the body parts, and organs, to each other and to the brain.

Nightguards and NTIs from a dental office can help relieve some of the symptoms of migraines without medication. Botox is also introduced in some cases to relieve the muscular tension contributing to the pain.

Supporting the adrenal, the thyroid, and the sex hormones, in an effort to support and back up each organ, will help tremendously. Short term sleep medication to help her body rest and heal may also help but then she should slowly get off the medication as her natural rhythm of sleep begins to revitalize itself.

SLEEP APNEA VERSUS SNORING

Sleep is greatly needed for healing, and positive moods towards life. Snoring can almost be harder on the spouse next to the offender than the person snoring themselves. However, if the person is actually suffering from sleep apnea, it can have huge adverse health effects on the person. Sleep apnea needs to be diagnosed properly through some type of a sleep study. You can go into a sleep study lab, and there are also take-home machines now as well. The treatment for most (once properly diagnosed) is a c pap machine. If one uses this method, it pushes positive pressure through the nose to keep the person using their diaphragm throughout the night breathing properly and not stopping to breath or jerking for a huge gasp of air. As you can imagine, gasping all night would not make for restful or healing sleep.

AUTOIMMUNE DISEASES

Autoimmune diseases are on a rise lately, probably due to the more inflammatory lifestyles we are all leading. Some of the most common ones you hear of are:

Syrgrons
Arthritis
Lupus
Phyhygoid
Pemphigus
Lichen Planus

Most of these autoimmune diseases affect some part of the endothelium of the body. The mouth can be a huge early symptom area for these diseases. A small biopsy from the cheek or offending area can reveal the root cause of the symptoms. With time signs begin to be more noticeable on the skin or deformation of the joints.

LIFE STYLE FACTORS

It is important to do what you can to remove stressors from your life. Stressors range from toxic people to typical relationships. We aren't suggesting you kick your spouse to the curb, but it may be time to set up some boundaries.

You may need a career change or at least a new position in the same field. You may need to have your debt restructured. These are all examples of stressors, but ultimately you have to look at your own life and make an honest assessment of what causes you stress.

Better sleep habits are a must! A bedtime by 10pm is ideal to take advantage of lower Cortisol levels—if you stay up too late and experience a "second wind," your cortisol levels have begun to rise again, not allowing your adrenals to get sufficient rest. A healthy sleep environment is achieved by a nice dark, cool room with either silence or white noise. Avoid the use of caffeine or alcohol at least four hours before bedtime.

Daily gentle exercise is an important factor. You should exercise as early in the day as possible for at least twenty to thirty minutes. This is not the time to start training for a marathon or a weight lifting competition. Gentle consistent exercise like swimming, walking or yoga is the key.

You need to do everything you can to restore your zest for life. When you learn how easy it is to feel happy and energetic again, you will be overwhelmed with laughter!

Research has found a positive medical link between laughter and the healthy function of blood vessels. In 2005 researchers at the University of Maryland Medical Center reported that laughter causes the inner lining of blood vessels, the endothelium, to dilate or expand enough to increase blood flow.

Drs. Michael Miller (University of Maryland) and William Fry (Stanford) theorize that beta-endorphin-like compounds released by the hypothalamus activate receptors on the endothelial surface to release nitric oxide, thereby resulting in dilation of vessels. Healthy good flowing blood keeps your blood pressure low and all organs getting what they need from the nutrients within our blood.

CUT 2 THE CHASE

Hormone Balance

Adrenals are the key to stress—Address the Stress! Remove some of the stressors from your life. You must consider supporting them with Vitamin B. By supporting your adrenals, they will help you support so many other important glands that produce more hormones.

It is important for both men and women to balance sex hormones of estrogen, testosterone and progesterone: as we age and experience stress, our sex hormones start to decline.

The decrease in sex hormones can tax the adrenals in two ways. First, because the adrenals are the backup system for sex hormones. Second, many inflammatory processes begin when the sex hormones decline, so the adrenals are required to produce more cortisol to counterbalance the inflammation.

Don't forget about checking your thyroid with a complete panel. Get the best look at how it is truly functioning with a comprehensive panel.

Nutrition

Nutritional supplements are a very important part of rebuilding the adrenals. Your protocol should include a Super B complex, Vitamin C, and fish oil. These will help rebuild glandular tissue as well as decrease inflammation.

It is very important that you be aware of any nutritional deficiencies that you may have. There are great micronutrient tests available that can tell you what your body is missing. The healthier you are in general, the less stress you will be putting on your adrenals.

As discussed in earlier chapters, foods can be very inflammatory, and testing for food sensitivities is important. Once you know what foods you are sensitive to and remove these foods from your diet, your body will be able to heal itself as well as absorb nutrients much better.

Remember that your digestive system makes up 60% of your immune system.

Purification
Chronic inflammation seems to be the root cause of so many diseases. Every day more and more research is being done on the links between them: our systems form a complicated relationship.

More comprehensive testing and evaluation of your body as a whole will reveal underlying causes of your unhealthy state. The answers you receive will act as a blueprint you can follow to your future health. Your family history is also crucial to identifying possible toxicity issues your family genetics may have. Use this information as a tool for purification options. Address your stress before it addresses you!

Neurons
Chiropractors devote their careers to keeping the communication pathways of your body open and clear. Make sure you do not have a curve in your highway of information. Get to the root source of your pain if you might be suffering from: Fibromyalgia, migraines, auto immune diseases, lupus, syrogrens, arthritis. All underlying causes connect back to chronic inflammatory diseases.

Sleep is essential. If you need to get the diagnoses right between snoring or sleep apnea, then do it. You won't get better until you get some rest.

Comprehensive testing will accurately show the assessment of your health and remove the guess work. Once you have the answers, it is easier to find solutions to make you feel better.

Saliva testing is our preferred method for testing most hormones, because it is simple and non-invasive and allows your practitioner to see what is bio-available (free floating) to be utilized by your tissues. Blood testing measures the levels of hormones that are attached to the red blood cells, so you can see trends of bio-availability.

Testing your main systems, function of the thyroid, adrenals, sex organs, and your food sensitivities seem to give the best chance to reveal your underlying health issues.

By making sure all of these areas or organs function optimally, you relieve stress off the adrenals and allow them time to recover, which empowers them to deal with STRESS better!

Chapter 9
How to Find Support

NOW IS THE TIME FOR THE RIGHT TREATMENT!

Do you ever wonder why you feel the way you do as you get older? Have you ever questioned or not fully understood a prescription or diagnosis your doctor has given you and its effect on your health? Are you seeking an alternative, preventive approach to, and an understanding of, your overall health and well-being? So are we.

Are you ready to address your stress?

You and your body deserve royal treatment – not just for one day, but every day! Now is the right time to access wellness and the best treatments possible, and reading this book has started you in the right direction to begin your journey.

PERSONALIZED MEDICINE

Over the last 20 years, medicine and healthcare providers have spread themselves out into specialties. There is nothing wrong with focusing in on one area and knowing it very well. After all, the body is a very complicated system.

However, your body is not multiple systems that just happen to work cohesively inside your body. It is a well thought-out machine of intertwined systems that only works well together in a healthy, well-cared for body.

We believe a shift in the way of thinking about healthcare is coming or is needed. We believe you have to go back to the basics! Some are now calling this shift "personalized medicine."

IT'S NOT JUST GETTING OLDER

When you feel bad or get sick, you often think you feel that way just because you are getting older.

That is not always the case! Sometimes, it is because you are not caring for your body the way you should. Deep down we all know this, it is just hard to admit. You think you will make it through anything and your body will endure anything you do to it. Your body begins to break down naturally with age, but the truth of the matter is that if you abuse your system long enough, it will begin to break down much faster than anticipated.

Sad to say, but once you feel bad for so long, you don't remember what is was like to feel good. Therefore, you lose motivation to get back to that happy, healthy place again.

TAKE CONTROL OF YOUR OWN HEALTH

Only you can truly control your own health—you have to address your stress! No magic drug that a doctor prescribes can give you back a healthy body.

Therefore, the time is now to get the right treatment. It is your ultimate responsibility to educate yourself and help your doctors or specialists take better care of you. We challenge you to get a friend, family member or co-worker and encourage each other to feel better. Find a doctor, dentist, or other healthcare provider that is willing to help you live your best life again.

The latest trend in healthcare is focused on patients taking control of their health and helping guide their doctors in their care.

Patients are becoming increasingly wary of the overuse of drugs and surgery and are seeking a more conservative and holistic approach.

THE BEST ANSWER TO HEALTH CARE REFORM – YOU!

Want to save money? Want to decrease health care spending? It is up to you! **GET HEALTHY!!!!**

A recent Gallup/American Health Poll says the first five health concerns are:

- Staying free from disease
- Avoiding smoking
- Living with clean air and pure water
- Having a positive outlook on life
- Having someone to love

The World Health Organization describes health as a state of complete physical, mental and social well-being. The bad news is that we are far from that statement being true in our society. In fact, chronic degenerative diseases consume 80% of healthcare dollars for conditions that are mostly preventable.

Both public and private payers are increasingly aware of the rising costs of chronic conditions. 10% of patients account for 70% of medical expenditures in the Medicare program.

Another significant fact is that 80% of people's improved health has nothing to do with health care providers; it has to do with what the patients do to improve their own situation.

Cardiovascular disease and cancer are the most common and costly conditions in the western world. Cardiovascular disease is largely attributed to poor diet, alcohol, smoking, hormone deficiencies, and no regular exercise. Most cancers can be prevented by adhering to a healthy diet, proper nutrition, hormone balance, and lifestyle modifications. Remember: 80% of patients' improvement of health falls solely on their personal actions to get their own health and well-being under control.

OUR BODIES ARE A CLOSED CIRCUIT COMPUTER BOARD

Your body is a closed system. If one aspect is out of whack, then the other systems have to try and make up for the deficiency. This might be okay for some time in some cases, but add another system out of sync or two or three more and before you know it, you feel awful and you don't know why.

You get frustrated because you just want to feel better. That prescription promising to fix all of your problems sounds so appealing and easy, so you get it and take it faithfully because it is the answer to your prayers. But is it really?

May we suggest that you keep educating yourself and see if there might be another way to approach the situation? If there were a way to possibly improve your overall health and well-being without a drug, wouldn't that be worth discovering?

In the past, only the elite could access the best health care and wellness opportunities. Now is the time you that you can begin to access this type of care for yourself. Now is the time you for you to be treated like a queen – like royalty. And so, your highness, let's get started.

CUT 2 THE CHASE

We hope you have decided that you are worthy of living your best life and that now is the right time for the right treatment. Support systems are in place to help you locate a health care provider or locate a virtual consultation to get the guidance you need. Remember: you are your best resource. Nobody knows or understands your body better than you do. In this era of personalized health care, you can and should be in charge of the decisions about how you want to feel. Are you ready to address your stress?

Visit **www.relevancehealth.com** and you will find a support system in place. To set up a virtual consultation with a caring healthcare provider is as simple as a click of the mouse. On this site you will also find easy to understand public education about your health and many helpful links to other wonderful health focused sites.

Many find it a challenge to get answers to their issues and to find alternatives to a magic prescriptive pill that will make them feel better. This site supports you with answers that may include a comprehensive line of pharmaceutical grade supplements. You will no longer need to worry about the quality of your vitamins or hormones. We stand behind our products.

Chapter 10
Easy Reference
to Hormones and Organs

Feel blessed that you did not go to medical school and were not required to learn the brutal details of each organ, system and hormone of the entire body. Just imagine those final exams! The body is a miracle. It is a complex piece of machinery, with no one manual, as each of us is different and unique. It puts your computer hard drive to shame. We don't think you need to know everything about every organ, but you do need to have a reference place to understand what the organs and glands do, what they influence, where they are located and how they communicate with each other.

ORGANS

The following section will highlight each organ's location, primary responsibilities, and other organs or systems it influences or communicates with.

Adrenal Glands
- Located at the top of each kidney
- Produce cortisol and adrenalin, and DHEA, plus supplemental estradiol (E2), testosterone and progesterone in small amounts
- Support our bodies during stress
- Prolonged exposure to stressors can exhaust the adrenals, leaving them ill-equipped to

supplement sex hormones when ovaries are not producing as many of these hormones.
- These small, walnut-sized, but powerful glands are strategically located in the body to quickly receive information from the anterior pituitary. The adrenals are also in close proximity to critical organs that the adrenal hormones act upon, including the liver, pancreas, kidneys, and others. They are involved in regulating virtually every aspect of bodily function.

Fat cells
- Located throughout the body, primarily in the abdomen, hips and thighs
- Produce the precursors to many hormones, plus E1 (estrogen)

Ovaries
- Located in the lower abdominal/pelvic area
- Produce estrogens, progesterone and testosterone
- During cycles when ovulation fails, little or no progesterone is produced
- After a woman's supply of eggs runs out (prior to menopause), the production of estrogen declines dramatically and almost no progesterone is produced.

Pancreas
- Located behind the stomach
- Produces insulin and other blood-sugar regulating substances

Pituitary Gland
- Located behind the brain, just above the roof of the mouth

- Produces LH (luteinizing hormone), FSH (follicle stimulating hormone) and other regulating hormones

Thyroid Gland
- A butterfly-shaped gland located at the base of the neck
- Produces thyroid hormones

Pineal Gland
- Located at the base of the brain
- Produces melatonin to manage circadian rhythms

Hypothalamus Gland
- Located in the brain
- Maintains homeostasis of hormones in the body

HORMONES

The following section will briefly highlight each hormone for easy reference.

Cortisol is the main hormone that directs immune function and is secreted in response to every day stressors. Its levels are tremendously valuable in assessing overall health. It is produced by the adrenal gland and works closely with adrenaline.

Adrenaline/ Epinephrine is the main hormone along with cortisol that releases energy for the flight or fight response. It narrows blood vessels, increases heart rate, opens airways, and decreases inflammation.

Aldosterone is produced by the adrenal glands and helps to maintain blood pressure by controlling fluid balance.

DHEA is produced by the adrenal glands. It supports brain function and produces testosterone.

Estrogen is categorized into several forms (E1/Estrone, E2/Estradiol, E3/Estriol), but collectively they function to develop female traits. Estrogen also slows bone loss, stimulates cell division, maintains tissue elasticity, reduces muscle mass, retains fluid, maintains heart health, supports brain function, and promotes a pleasant mood. Estrogen is produced by ovaries and fat cells. There is much confusion regarding estrogen supplementation, with cancer causing a concern due to the stimulation of advanced cellular division.

Endorphins promote a feeling of wellbeing and reduce pain and are produced by the pituitary and the hypothalamus.

FSH is a follicle-stimulating hormone produced by the anterior pituitary. The main responsibility of FSH is to mature eggs and sperm.

Gastrin is produced by the G cells and assists in the release of stomach acid.

Glucose (Blood Sugar) provides energy for virtually all cells.

Growth Hormone's main function is to stimulate growth and cell division. It also repairs tissue, maintains bone, brain, muscle, skin, hair, and nails.

Insulin is produced by the pancreas. The main function of insulin is to regulate blood sugar and produce triglycerides.

Leptin decreases appetite, increases metabolism and is produced by our fat cells.

Melatonin is the key to your circadian rhythm. Its main responsibility is to promote REM sleep.

Oxytocin is a key hormone for child birth in women. Oxytocin stimulates bonding emotions, the release of breast milk, and triggers contractions in the cervix.

Parathyroid supports bone and is essential in activating vitamin D production.

Progesterone is a key factor in pregnancy. It softens the uterine lining to prepare your body to have a period, enabling reproduction. Progesterone also is key in balancing the effects of estrogen. It builds bone and muscle, promotes fat burning, stabilizes blood sugar, supports the thyroid, elevates the mood, enhances brain function, and creates a sex drive.

Prolactin is produced by the pituitary gland. It promotes the feeling of satisfaction after sex and the production of breast milk.

Serotonin is a key player in sleep. It also supports the appetite and controls the mood. Serotonin is produced in the gastrointestinal tract and the central nervous system.

Testosterone is key to developing male traits. It promotes assertiveness, elevates the mood, maintains heart and brain function, and builds bone and muscle.

Testosterone is produced in the ovaries and in the testicles.

Thyroid hormones like T3 and T4 are produced by the thyroid gland. Major responsibilities of the thyroid are the control of metabolism and body temperature.

TSH (Thyroid-stimulating hormone) triggers the release of thyroid hormones. TSH is not produced by the thyroid; the pituitary gland actually produces TSH as a feed-back loop to the production of thyroid hormones.

Lightning Source UK Ltd.
Milton Keynes UK
UKOW06f1954291015

261703UK00015B/493/P

9 781457 507014